PERSONAL HISTORY & HEALTH

The Midtown
Longitudinal Study
1954 - 1974

PERSONAL HISTORY & HEALTH

Leo Srole
Ernest Joel Millman

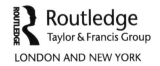 Routledge
Taylor & Francis Group

LONDON AND NEW YORK

First published 1998 by Transaction Publishers

Published 2017 by Routledge
2 Park Square, Milton Park, Abingdon, Oxon OX14 4RN
711 Third Avenue, New York, NY 10017, USA

First issued in paperback 2018

Routledge is an imprint of the Taylor & Francis Group, an informa business

Library of Congress Catalog Number: 97-26145

Library of Congress Cataloging-in-Publication Data

Srole, Leo.
    Personal history and health : the Midtown Longitudinal Study, 1954–1974 / Leo Srole and Ernest Joel Millman.
        p. cm.
    Includes bibliographical references and index.
    ISBN 1-56000-325-1 (alk. paper)
    1. Mental health—United States—Longitudinal studies. 2. Mental health—United States—Longitudinal studies. 3. Mental illness—Forecasting—Longitudinal studies. I. Millman, Ernest Joel. II. Title.
RA790.6.S7   1997
362.2'0422—dc21   97-26145
                                                                    CIP

ISBN 13: 978-1-138-51304-4 (pbk)
ISBN 13: 978-1-56000-325-0 (hbk)

Contents

Preface

Without the strong and unwavering support of Esther Srole, wife of the late senior author, the present work would have been quite impossible. The equally valuable support of my wife, Ellen F. Pepperberg Millman is lovingly acknowledged. Finally this work might never have been published as one monograph, presenting the totality of the Midtown Longitudinal Study findings regarding the life-span predictors of mental health and other outcomes, without the interest and support of Irving Louis Horowitz.

This work represents the late Leo Srole's final perspectives on adult mental health. As was characteristic of him, it is exploratory, not confirmatory; it raises questions, and does not declare conclusions. Through this work Leo completes his pioneering of the exploration of social age and adult mental health, in particular as the character of social age might have differed for the women and men of the Midtown Longitudinal Study. His description of how the Midtown panel was assembled in 1974 after a twenty year hiatus is an invaluable contribution to longitudinal research.

The title of the monograph, *Personal History and Health*, reflects the nature of most of the research analyses described here, in which the unit of analysis was the individual Midtowner. Such group characteristics as Gender and Generation are represented in these analyses as characteristics of the person, as are such outcomes as mental health and history of somatic disorders.

During the approximately three decades of the Midtown Longitudinal Study, from inception to present, Leo was joined by a host of research collaborators. Many predated my collaboration with Leo, which began in 1976. They are acknowledged in the published reports from the Midtown Longitudinal Study in which they participated. (See the bibliographies of chapters 1–5.)

Leo's associates from 1976 on were also mine, whom I acknowledge here:

Leo Srole, Ph.D. himself provided me with the opportunity to enjoy my first publication, and endorsed the methodical use of path analysis which structures much of this monograph. His emphasis on discovering *predictors* of adult mental health rather than speculating on cause-and-effect defined what was and what was not possible to achieve with the Midtown Longitudinal Study data set.

The late Anita K. Fischer contributed in countless ways to Leo's work. Her focus on gender differences in mental health became a major impetus of this study.

Three uniquely valuable friends and colleagues from the Teachers College, Columbia University, Social Psychology Program (which no longer enjoys an independent existence) made my participation in the Midtown Longitudinal Study possible, in many ways: Janos Marton, Ph.D. brought me to Leo's attention in 1976, when the study team needed an additional member to implement the life-span path analyses of mental health projected but, until then, never implemented. I had intensively studied path analysis during my graduate program years and had planned to use path analysis in my dissertation, which was underway at the time. Janos has continued to be a staunch friend and an invaluable resource to me through the years. He now directs the Living Museum at Creedmoor Psychiatric Center, in Queens Village, New York. Michael Freund, Ph.D. showed me the ropes concerning the construction and maintenance of large SPSS data archives. He expertly checked my construction of the indices used in the first life-span path analyses and provided friendly support for my efforts during the first three years of my participation in the Midtown Longitudinal Study. Most importantly, Michael worked with his friend Janos to assist Leo in bringing to its final state the computer simulation of the 1954 Psychiatrists' Ratings of mental health, which yielded the primary outcome variable of this study. Michael now edits the weekend edition of the primary liberal newspaper of Austria. Jackson Kytle, Ph.D. constructed the index of Social Network Density. For fifteen months I was employed by him at Antioch University, during which time we worked together on a number of scholarly essays. Jack continues to pursue a career which combines educational administration with social scientific and philosophical pursuits.

Five additional, and most recent, associates of ours remain to be acknowledged. Barry Gurland, M.D., Sidney Katz, Professor of Psychiatry and Director of the Stroud Center for Study of Quality of Life of Columbia University, and principal investigator of numerous research projects, has been a strong supporter of this study for the past two decades. Lirio Covey, Ph.D. constructed this study's 1974 Occupational Level index, a very challenging task. She has been honored as an outstanding research scientist at New York State Psychiatric Institute. James L. Curtis, M.D., Clinical Professor of Psychiatry, Columbia University and Director of Psychiatry, Harlem Hospital Center, has been my employer since 1984 and has been warmly supportive in many ways of my efforts in completing this study. He and all of his clinical colleagues in the Department of Psychiatry have been my mentors in public mental health since 1984. Elmer L. Struening, Ph.D., Director of the Epidemiology of Mental Disorders Research Department, New York State Psychiatric Institute, graciously extended his computer privileges to me so that the final analyses could be computed. "Moose" was a good friend of Leo and Esther, and a colleague of Leo's in the Psychiatric Epidemiology Training Program, Division of Epidemiology, School of Public Health, Columbia University. An expert on program evaluation research of national stature whose most recent of many honors was a celebratory evening at the American Public Health Association's convention in October 1996, he has closely collaborated with James Curtis and me on a follow-up study of intensive case management for discharged psychiatric inpatients. Leo Srole carefully documented all of the sources of support for this study (e.g., in Srole 1980), as follows: The Midtown Longitudinal Study in its first stage (1952–1959) was sponsored by the Cornell Medical College and supported by grants from the National Institute of Mental Health (NIMH no. M515) to the late Thomas A. C. Rennie, M.D., professor of psychiatry, Cornell University Medical College. Supplementary support was acknowledged from the Grant Foundation, the Rockefeller Brothers Fund, the Milbank Foundation, the Littauer Foundation and the Samuel Rubin Foundation. Access to the Midtown I data bank was made possible through the cooperation of Stanley Michael, M.D., and Robert Michels, M.D., Chairman, Cornell Department of Psychiatry. Special acknowledgements of a number of consultants were specified, including Louis Linn, M.D., Jean Endicott, Ph.D, Steven M. Cohen, Ph.D., Donald Treiman, Ph.D., Richard Remington, M.D., W. Edwards Deming, Ph.D., Robert Markush, M.D., Ben Locke, M.S., and Shirley Reff-Margolis, Ph.D., of the NIMH Center for Epidemiological Studies. In its second stage (1972–1982) the Study was first sponsored by the New York State Psychiatric Institute and Columbia College of Physicians and Surgeons, Department of Psychiatry, chaired by Drs. Lawrence C. Kolb, Sidney Malitz, Edward J. Sachar, and most recently John M. Oldham. Its operational grants were from the NIMH Center for Epidemiological Studies (MH no.13369) and the Foundation's Fund for Research, Fritz Redlich, M.D., President, with Leo Srole as Principal Investigator. Data analyses and reports through 31 May 1981 were supported under grant 32794 from the NIMH Center for Epidemiological Studies and Center for Aging Studies.

We also acknowledge, as users of the New York State Psychiatric Institute's computer facility, the support of Mental Health Research Center Grant MH 39896 from the National Institute of Mental Health.

The Statistical Appendices

When the late Leo Srole and Anita Fischer put together the research design and funding proposals for the Midtown Longitudinal Study, they selected the statistical methods of multiple correlation and regression analysis as the means to explore the basic ideas of this study. However Leo was always uncomfortable with the extensive presentation of statistical tables and figures which these methods entail. In the first presentation of our research on long-term perspectives on adult mental health (Fischer et al. 1979) we chose to relegate the tables and figures to an appendix so that the reader could receive an uninterrupted narrative. This approach has also been taken in this, Leo Srole's final presentation of this study. All of the statistical explanations, details, figures, and tables have been placed in a set of Statistical Appendices. Statistically sophisticated readers who would like to refer to these materials, and perhaps critically evaluate their use and interpretation in this monograph, may obtain them from University Microfilms, Inc. To order, either telephone University Microfilms at 1-800-521-0600 or fax at 1-313-665-5022, and request manuscript LD03613.

References

Fischer, Anita K., Janos Marton, Ernest J. Millman, and Leo Srole. 1979. "Long-range influences on adult mental health: The Midtown Manhattan Longitudinal Study, 1954–1974," in *Research in Community and Mental Health, Vol. 1*, edited by Roberta G. Simmons, 305–33. Greenwich, CT: JAI Press.

Srole, Leo with Anita Kassen Fischer. "The Midtown Manhattan Longitudinal Study vs. 'The Mental Paradise Lost' Doctrine." *Archives of General Psychiatry* 37 (February 1980): 209–21.

1

Introduction

Prelude: A Tale of Two Towns

Throughout recorded history scientists, philosophers, and storytellers have sought to understand how it is that their fellows can appear to remain the same while at the same time changing all the while. Behavioral scientists have been trying to catch up with the novelists and playwrights who have explored and exposed the dramatic conflicts between human stability and change. The present authors are among the relatively few behavioral scientists who have chosen to follow the progress of a large cohort of people, in this case as they experienced a considerable portion of their adult lives from when they were first studied in 1954 to when they were reinterviewed twenty years later, in 1974.

The rare narrative to be related about these people can best be introduced by noting several of its similarities with the story line of one of the most popular American plays of the twentieth century, *Our Town*, written by Thornton Wilder on the eve of World War II. Although the two works will have obvious divergences, the central convergence is that each sweeps us into an identified social landscape, an entire community, its cast of local characters enlisted to speak for their neighbors.

Mr. Wilder's imaginary "Grover's Corners" is a settlement with 2,642 inhabitants. The community in which our cohort lived when we[1] first made their acquaintance, in 1954, was found teeming with life in a well delineated residential section of New York City, one we called "Midtown." At our arrival, some 172,275 people resided in Midtown. In the light of their contrasting numbers, the two communities could appropriately have been called "Small Town" and "Big Town" respectively, both located in the same region of the United States that the Census Bureau labels "The Northeast." By 1974 only about one in five of this cohort still lived at their original address in Midtown. About an additional one in five had remained in Manhattan, while about one in

1

five had moved to the other boroughs of New York City. The remaining two-fifths lived outside of New York City in 1974. Although the cohort was geographically dispersed by the end of the third quarter of the twentieth century, they all had shared the experience of residing in Midtown at midcentury and of being a part of the Midtown study.

The printed program of a play usually specifies the historical period on which its curtains open. The actions in the two towns are set several generations apart: One takes place in the early years of this century, the other during the century's third quarter, with Grover's Corners reflecting the rural nature of the region in its town, and Midtown the prevailing urbanism of a half century later. Despite these differences in historical period and geography, the two works have a common agenda, namely one of following their separate casts across a rather sizeable span of time—Grover's Corners for the twelve years 1901–1913, in Midtown for the twenty years 1954–1974.

That agenda, involving a modern kind of "Pilgrim's Progress," is to capture and describe in a summary way, as with a time-lapse camera, the final state of the characters, after all of the factors which produce continuity or change in people's lives have occurred. Here the two enterprises, so different in how they express their reports on peoples' lives, converge on common narrative ground.

Wilder raises his community above the particular details of a conventional locale, by giving it the following inclusive postal address: "Grover's Corners, New Hampshire, the United States of America, Western Hemisphere, Earth, the Solar System, the Universe, the Mind of God."

Although as scientists studying a particular group of people in a limited time period we cannot begin to picture such an all-embracing cosmos, we do seek to understand the larger significance of the Midtown cohort who have been observed in considerable detail, at about the beginning and ending of the third quarter of the twentieth century, through the trained eyes of behavioral scientists. Although Wilder's perceptions were those of the imaginatively expressive artist, there is a parallel between his self-chosen role, vis-à-vis his characters, and our own vis-à-vis our subjects.

The story line of *Our Town* is carried primarily by an unusual character, one seemingly on a higher level than that of the townspeople. He combines the roles of narrator, commentator and play-director-within-the-play, labelled by Wilder as "STAGE MANAGER." (Capitalization follows the play's script; "SM" hereafter is our acronym for him.) SM's part is largely monologue, addressed to the audience, weaving through the spoken lines of the interacting town characters. What comes through early on is SM's implicit image of himself as an outsider observing the life of the town, in an approximation of the role of the visiting behavioral scientist. For example he confides to his audience, "We want a little more information about the town, kind of a scientific account you might say. So, I've asked Professor Willard of our State University to sketch a few details..." Echoing SM one character remarks, "The day wouldn't come when I wouldn't want to know everything that is happening here."

After the professor has reported some of that locality's features, SM calls on "Mr. Webb," editor of the weekly *Sentinel*, who among other things offers a miniature sociodemographic profile of the town, as follows (we quote Webb verbatim): "We're lower middle class, sprinkling of professional men...ten percent illiterate laborers...Religiously, we're eighty-five percent Protestants, twelve percent Catholics, rest indifferent." He also might have confirmed thus far that in racial composition Grover's Corners is almost entirely white.

Related Midtown details will be reported presently, but other parallels in the descriptive functions of SM and the present authors deserve prior mention. SM situates Grover's Corners with a seemingly exact latitude and longitude, although on a map that conjunction falls well offshore in the Atlantic. On Midtown's part such precision is hardly necessary, for it is a conspicuous district on an island which commands the great harbor where the mouth of the Hudson River opens on the Atlantic. Midtown is one of the island's larger residential quarters, tagged by two postal zip numbers and housing at mid-century a white population some sixty-five times bigger than that reported for Grover's Corners.

Playwright Wilder peoples his stage with 23 characters of ages ranging from adolescent to middle age, accounting for 9 per 1,000 of the village's residents. On the other hand the Midtown study team, of which the senior author was a principal member, originally focussed almost its entire attention on Midtown's midlife cohort, aged 20 to 59, numbering approximately 110,000 inhabitants in 1954.

As its first task, through an average interview lasting about two hours, the Midtown study team collected the confidential testimony of a mathematically randomized, demographically representative cross-section sample of 1,660 of these individuals, accounting for 15 per 1,000 of their total peers of like age.

SM literally "manages" the on-stage appearances of his cast ensemble, and either questions them informally, as he did with the editor and the professor, or temporarily leaves the stage for them to reveal themselves with close role partners in the play.

For the Midtown sample of adults the study team prepared a long and painstakingly designed schedule of questions to obtain comparable kinds of personal information from all 1,660 of them. This "answer completion" format helped each Midtowner to briefly tell their life history in a way that could be compared with the life histories of the other subjects. Staff interviewers were the Team's personal surrogates in guiding subjects' testimony on important facets of their lives, past and present, and also its "eyes" in recording observations about each individual's behavior and feelings during the long session. Taken altogether, what we gathered added up to a confidential collective autobiography.

The Midtown Study was originally expected to yield the equivalent of a one-sitting, composite group portrait of the sample, and was so reported in a large series of journal articles, doctoral dissertations and two monographs, one of the latter in three editions.[2]

The volume of such publications cannot remotely compare with the post-1938 multiple editions of *Our Town* within book covers, and thousands of live productions by amateur, "little theater" and professional companies in towns and cities as far abroad as the Soviet Union and China, with additional performances seen by millions of movie and television viewers. Thornton Wilder seems to have anticipated that his drama would become an enduring theatrical classic all over the world.

We do not imply any comparison when we add that the Midtown publication record mentioned is as yet incomplete. From the start the latter had been planned and conducted to be complete in itself, in effect a one-act report. As pioneers on the new research frontier beginning after World War II, carrying out one of the largest undertakings of its kind up to that time, the Midtown study team did not remotely conceive the possibility of a study to follow directly in its footsteps.

However as director of the Midtown field staff, the senior author had monitored the incoming interviewing documents for quality control purposes. In the process he discovered that the sampled subjects' individual personalities were vividly displayed in their recorded testimony, making him want to know them more fully.

To a closing letter of appreciation sent to all interviewed subjects, some had replied with holiday greeting cards bearing additional family and personal news. He always answered these notes, which in turn were occasionally followed by other two-way communications, both written and by telephone.[3]

As a result, while writing the flagship volume of the 1954 study the senior author realized that he had become inextricably involved with the 1,660 subjects.[4] Inevitably, his thoughts returned to them with the insistent question: How have their further life experiences affected them, as they aged biologically to the accompaniment of long-range changes in their national, local and family settings?

To answer this question an additional follow-up study would be needed. Supporting such a study were two larger trends: First was the appearance of several follow-up investigations of broadly parallel kinds; these had studied life-course ups-and-downs as a process that engages all of us in the role of protagonists.[5] Second, in the early-1960's Congressional and academic leaders began to recognize their need for a national monitoring program to chart social trends on a regular basis. They felt the need for "means by which our society can assess where we are now and where we have been, and provide a basis of anticipation—rather than prediction—of where we are going in a number of areas critical to our national welfare...Our highly developed national system of economic indicators, which allows us to measure the state of our economy in considerable detail, needs to be supplemented with information on the state of our society in those areas not...within the professional domain of the economist."[6]

Emphasizing the urgency of this need were the consequences of the assassinations of several national political leaders, leaving many people with a sense of national and personal dislocation, as well as producing economic disruptions and even riots. The Midtown study of a large, general urban population, which gave signs of varying considerably in individual well-being, had been conducted in a relatively calm year during the early 1950's. Given the 1954 battery of intensive information available for replication, it therefore could conveniently lend itself to conversion into a baseline for studying the subsequent, cumulative impacts of the period 1954–1974 on the Midtowners.

This was a unique and exciting opportunity: Never before had any scientist been able to assemble so extensive a body of intimate details of the lives of so large and representative a sample population, to be individually followed-up after two decades, a period often taken to define a "generation."[7] We could not anticipate, however, that this would be so tumultuous and disorderly a period, which ran from Eisenhower's early White House years through the Vietnam period to the Watergate scandal, ending with the very last day of Nixon's presidency; these historical developments made the follow-up study all the more valuable.

With these thrilling prospects and a new staff, the senior author turned to designing a follow-up investigation—not previously contemplated—as a climatic second act, the two to be designated Midtown I and II (also known as MHIM1 and MHIM2). Of course the latter demanded that we locate and reinterview as many of the 1,660 Midtowners as could be found after an interval of twenty years. The biggest of our unknown study factors, we shall tell the story of this unplanned "needles in the haystack" search in the following chapter.

In terms similar to those of the theater, our original Midtowners were actors on the continuously moving, arena-sized stage of Manhattan. After 1954 several hundred died; several hundred had moved to other stages in New York City; other hundreds were resettled in surrounding counties, in forty states on the continent and in twelve far-flung countries abroad; and several hundred more had completely disappeared. Thus in 1954 about three-quarters of the Midtowners had been immigrants from sites varying distances beyond New York City and national boundaries; by 1974 some three-fifths of those located alive resided outside of Midtown.

However by 1974 a majority of 858 were located alive and could be reinterviewed. Some 163 could not or chose not to be reinterviewed. The remaining 695 people, now aged 40 to 79, are our players in the Study's second act, observed and reinterviewed in their current residences for systematic comparison both with themselves twenty years younger, and with peers then and now.[8]

The setting of the last act of *Our Town* is the local cemetery. Ten chairs, serving as prop grave stones, are occupied by actors representing the dead beneath those markers. Into their midst file the mourners in a burial cortege. To the previous act's theme of "Love and Marriage" this act provides the closure of mortality and intimations of the life beyond.

It is not often that a playwright makes the purposes of his play explicit in the body of the work, as does Thornton Wilder in *Our Town*. In its first act SM relates that construction has begun of a new bank building, which will incorporate a cornerstone for a time capsule of selected documents, including copies (here listed in his own sequence) of "The *New York Times*, the local newspaper, the Bible, the Constitution of the United States, a book of Shakespeare, and one contemporary play." As explanation for the choice of that particular drama, SM tells us: "Y'know...in Greece and Rome, all we know about the *real* life of the people is what we can piece together out of the joking poems and the comedies they wrote for their theater back then...so I'm going to have a copy of this play [i.e., *Our Town*] put in the cornerstone...so people a thousand years from now—this is the way we were in the provinces north of New York at the beginning of the twentieth century. This is the way we were; in our growing up and in our marrying and in our living and dying."

Wilder seems to be saying that his play is addressed to audiences of two very separate eras. For people living a thousand years in the future, the drama is projected as a testimonial record, analogous perhaps to the Dead Sea Scrolls speaking for an ancient settlement that called itself "The Community of Qumran." For us, Wilder's contemporaries, *Our Town* is a parable about the elementary, commonplace beats of the clock of life, disrupted at irregular intervals by the gains and losses of attachments that accompany the passage of every human from birth to burial and beyond. For the reader approaching the closing curtain of the century, the book now in hand weaves a similar, more intricately laced, tapestry.

Two decades after the opening of *Our Town* on Broadway, the author commented that the play "is an attempt to find a value above all price for the smallest events of our life..." In the present book we follow Mr. Wilder's example in fixing on one particular "value above all price," namely that of health and well-being, in a representative company of big towners (past and for the most part present)—and in the final reckoning, perhaps, that of All Towners in the twilight years of their common century.

Midtown Unveiled

A passing bird's-eye view of Midtown has been rendered in comparison to Grover's Corners. The purpose of this longitudinal study is to assess the degree to which Midtowners changed biologically, socially and psychologically over the twenty years, beginning in 1954, and to develop a long-range life-span perspective on those changes. We also intend to explore the extent to which changes over the twenty years resemble the differences between two groups of Midtowners, that is those who were 40 to 59 in 1954 and those who were 40 to 59 in 1974. By comparing the differences associated with twenty years of biological aging with those associated with being a part of the 40 to 59 generation either twenty years sooner or later (that is in 1954 or in 1974) we may discover the extent to which differences among Midtowners which seemingly are due to biological "age" are actually due to social "age," that is the Midtowners' membership in one versus another Generation. We shall also explore the extent to which the differences associated with either biological or social "age" are the same or different for Midtown women and men. To doubly protect their original anonymity we have always kept the identity of their area of residence under the cloak of a shielding code name.

However during the intervening decades most of our reinterviewed Midtowners have moved out of the Study area to new residences, some as far away as other countries. Nevertheless for the sake of narrative continuity between studies I and II we retain their original designation as Midtowners.

Another development has been persuasive in our decision to drop the cloak. Beginning in the late 1940s a backlog of commercial construction planned for Manhattan's Central Business district, but postponed due to World War II, began to be built, at an increasing pace during the subsequent four decades. This resulted in a tidal wave of demand for residential housing in the adjoining areas, which impacted most forcefully on Midtown's pre-WWI tenement rows, many of which have since been remodelled or replaced by high-rent skyscraper apartments. For many New Yorkers, in particular, the long chain of reactions triggered by this massive upgrading process, often referred to as "Urban Renewal," had the dislocating effect of an earthquake, exactly centering on the Midtown study area.

Thus we may now reveal its identity, beginning with an outline of its boundaries.[9] Starting with the district to its north, East Harlem in ethnic and socioeconomic coloration was markedly different from the Midtown population, 99 percent white in 1954, such that their shared 96th Street border has long been characterized as "a Ghetto Wall," shrinking the normal Manhattan north-south cross-flow of vehicular and pedestrian traffic to trickles.[10]

At the opposite border, on a workday to cross vehicle-jammed 59th Street from the south is to transit from one of the nation's biggest and busiest commercial areas into a quiet retreat of apartment "cliff dwellings" and four-story walk-up brownstone houses.

With the confining East River at another of its sides, three of the borders represent what urban sociologists call "natural boundaries," of a type that sharply cut off a city section from its contrasting surroundings.

The Park Avenue border, on the other hand, separates the Study area from a two-block corridor fronting on Central Park that shelters the largest, most homogeneous concentration of residential wealth in all of New York City, and in local weekly newspapers is sometimes perceived as a "Silk Stocking Strip," by comparison with the far more diversified six-block area stretching beyond Park Avenue to the East River.

All in all, with a surface space of some 1.4 square miles, a population density of 123,000 inhabitants per square mile, conspicuous sociocultural diversity, and a considerable variety of specialized shopping outlets and service agencies, the Study area was a compact and partially self-contained residential district, with an identity that is often inclusively tagged in the press as "the Upper East Side." Set on what has been called a "tight little island," it was sociologically a quasi-insular community, consisting of loosely differentiated neighborhoods.[11]

Midtown has been now defined as a distinct geographical entity, to which we have applied the description "community." The latter is a general term that accommodates a wide variety of human groupings, ranging from, at minimum, a face-to-face neighborhood, to a worldwide "community of nations," that is, President Bush's "New World Order." Here we are using the word's lesser sense of any population whose members are inhabitants of a limited physical locale, one that is either legally incorporated within specified boundaries, or is a named, bounded part of such an incorporated entity.

As an enormously complex but relevant example, Manhattan, up to 1898, was the incorporated "City of New York." After that date it was legally renamed "County of New York" (alternatively the "Borough of Manhattan") within the merged five-borough body of Greater New York.[12] Thus our study area qualifies, under the above definition, as a named section of the island of Manhattan that is officially an incorporated county.[13]

Why Midtown?

We must next address the reader's plausible question: Why, at the very start of the Study, was Midtown, among all possible areas, chosen for an intensive public health survey? Worthy of brief review are three separate considerations that influenced the choice.

1. The National Institute of Mental Health (NIMH) was set up to fund research and personnel training programs in its field, and with a recognition that community investigations were necessary to support its public health objectives.[14] To this end, it was assumed that for com-

parative purposes a variety of community types would have to be surveyed. In fact communities had long been classified by the size of their populations, ranging from the village to the metropolis.

These categories of community were especially important for public health purposes, because through the entirety of Western history they had been associated with sharp contrasts in the frequencies of a variety of human afflictions. The correlation formula ran something like this: The bigger and denser the settlement the more prevalent these disorders appeared to be. In this light, exploration of a big city presented itself as a top priority.

2. Coincidentally, among the first proposals to conduct an epidemiological community study was that submitted to NIMH by the prominent social psychiatrist Dr. Thomas A.C. Rennie. Especially favoring approval of his application were the facts that he was a senior professor in the Cornell Medical College and clinical associate of the New York Hospital; both institutions are parts of a major medical complex based at the eastern edge of the Midtown Study area.

As a further advantage, office quarters for the researchers were offered in the Hospital, such that from 1952 to 1959 the Study team were almost daily observers of, and to some "extracurricular" extent participants in, the local scene. The study greatly profited both from its explicit identification with these two highly visible and eminent medical institutions, and from the senior researchers' formal and informal ties with local leaders, including clergymen, who helped obtain community approval of its research program of confidential interviews with a large sample of resident adults. To our knowledge, few other community studies managed, to the same extent, to mobilize invaluable long-term resident support for such personal explorations.

3. Published Census Bureau data of 1950 showed that the demographic composition of the population within the boundaries of Midtown was, at that time, a close approximation of the 1.2 million white, non-Puerto Rican residents of the borough of Manhattan.[15] In short, on demographic criteria the Midtowners were a reasonably representative cross-section of a much larger white population universe, one that stood at the summit of metropolitan America.

Stated in other words, the Midtown population was a community entity which had a more generalizable, scientific significance than its compact character might suggest, one that transcended its incidental, particular characteristics.

On all three of the above considerations, the choice of Midtown for a public health investigation was, so to speak, "a natural." This conclusion received seemingly unanimous support some years later in 1962, when *Mental Health in the Metropolis* was published, to the accompaniment of extraordinary coverage in the daily press, news magazines and professional journals. In none, so far as we know, was the choice of study area in any way challenged.

On the other hand, word-of-mouth criticism did ultimately reach us on the absence of African Americans in the otherwise socioculturally heterogeneous Midtown population. The criticism warrants an open reply in this sequel volume.

1. To have added African-Americans in numbers sufficient for statistical purposes would have required that the Study team break out of its limited budget, and to cross borders into a community entity of a rather contrasting type.

2. In retrospect, even with sufficient funds, some of the Study team, at least, would have been skeptical about its competence and visible acceptability to probe the intimacies of well-being in a highly ghettoized black population.[16]

3. In any case, it was a plausible hope that a Midtown-scale study of a metropolitan black community would in due course emerge, as indeed one did.[17]

Research Origins and Targets

The present study, MHIM2, originated in the Midtown I (MHIM1) Study. To view MHIM1 investigation in larger perspective, we must pause to review the historical circumstances that had impelled it, indeed had shaped it, and by extension had also shaped its follow-up successor. At the very least, then, such a rearview account will perhaps explain to the reader the motives for doing what we did; just as motives are indispensable to understanding a crime, so are they essential to comprehending the "why" of a research project.

MHIM1 was born out of the labor pangs of World War II. In particular we refer to the lessons America painfully learned after the shocks of Pearl Harbor in attempting, almost overnight, to mobilize the largest military machine in its history. Issues on the fitness of the conscripted manpower were later critically addressed in "The Ineffective Soldier" studies at Columbia University. For our purposes here, the main source of information is its monograph *The Lost Divisions* by Professor Ginzberg and his colleagues.[18]

Long before the end of the war, Ginzberg tells us,

> ...the first alarms were being sounded by those who had become acquainted with the mounting casualty figures which reflected soldiers' breaking down with one or another type of psychiatric disability.[19] These data were not released to the public for fear they would enable the enemy to glean useful information from them about the state of our manpower resources...
>
> Among the distinguished leaders of the psychiatric profession who sounded the alarm were many who had long suspected on the basis of their private practice that for every patient whom they saw there were ten others who, though in need of help, had never consulted a doctor. The war seemed to prove their point. [Other] scattered evidence pointed to the prevalence of mental illness in the American population...
>
> [When] the wartime restrictions on the release of official data were lifted...many startling facts and figures became available to the public for the first time.[20]

We need not unravel the extremely complicated administrative history behind those "startling" seven-digit totals of the number of selective service "rejections" and inductee "premature discharges" recorded for "physical, mental, emotional, and administrative reasons."

An early outgrowth of these revelations was Congressional establishment in 1948 of the National Institute of Mental Health as a new training, treatment and research funding arm of the U.S. Public Health Service. With the entire national population as its charge, one of the first items on the NIMH agenda was to sponsor investigations of various communities.

The initial series of such studies supported by NIMH were of two major types. One, in a tradition going back to the seventeenth century, was essentially a file count of admissions to mental institutions. This tradition reached its high-water mark in a study by two sociologists of 27,000 Chicago patients admitted for psychoses to state and county hospitals between the years 1922 and 1934.[21]

The second type of community investigation, first supported by NIMH in the early 1950s, was based on the recognition that the large wartime manpower pool called for examination had excluded individuals with psychiatric histories. Therefore, those militarily rejected or discharged on psychological grounds represented a sizeable, previously unidentified portion of the general population, warranting attention as an unrecognized public health problem. On this basis a series of community-wide face-to-face investigations of local people in "all walks of life" was needed.[22]

The Midtown Study, the largest of the first four of this type, was in effect an independent expedition to a new scientific frontier, that required a study team combining an assortment of professional skills never brought together before the War. First in order was psychiatry, the medical specialty serving patients labelled as mentally ill, and principally treated at that time in mental hospital settings isolated from their communities. Accordingly it was no accident that a senior professor of clinical psychiatry in the Cornell Medical College was funded by NIMH to become the director of the MHIM1 Team.

Because it focussed on a large community entity, the Study's second priority called for a social science specialist in community field research. With a background in social anthropology and experience in several of such pre-war American undertakings, the senior author was recruited to serve as the team's senior social scientist and full-time field director.

Added to the team in its early years, on a full-time, part-time, or consultant basis, were representatives of clinical psychology, cultural anthropology, biostatistics, and psychiatric social work. Joined with clinical psychiatry, this mixed group of representatives of autonomous disciplines, each with its own professional turf and vocabulary, were ultimately roped together under the rubric of "behavioral science" into a study team.[23]

The spurring lesson of wartime examinations of military-age men, the construction of a powerful new psychiatric agency in the federal government, the pressure of making diverse individual specialists into a team, the mandate to persuade community residents in some numbers to accept personal interviews, and the implicit expectation that the study would yield guidelines for expanding and reorganizing psychiatric services all converged to create an unusually urgent atmosphere that enveloped the newly born MHIM1 as one of the first of its kind.

It was in this pressing atmosphere that the MHIM1 research staff began a process of hammering out a series of state-of-the-art procedural decisions. For the study team to investigate the entire general population of Midtown was not remotely possible. And it was rendered unnecessary by the then recent invention of probability sampling, a statistical technology for systematic, objective selection of a relatively small number of subjects from an overarching population of research interest, who would comprise a representative cross section in miniature of that population (with a known, tolerably small margin of error).[24]

As a first step, the study team reduced Midtown's birth to late geriatric age range by selecting men and women in the career-involved midlife age range between 20 and 59 years, bringing down its eligible total from 172,000 to about 110,000. From the latter the team next drew 1,660 representative subjects. These were engaged by the team in home interviews conducted by especially trained New York professionals in such fields as psychology, social work, sociology, and anthropology.

To standardize the interviews from subject to subject, senior Study staff constructed a meticulously worded sequence of questions addressed to their 1,660 respondent-interviewees. The contents of those questions can be visualized as a series of concentric circles that resemble a rifle-practice target. The center of the target was fixed on the concept of "health," one of the most loosely and commonly used words in the language, occupying as well a special position in Western thought. The degree to which it is ever in our thoughts and speech is suggested by the almost universal greeting of two people familiar with each other, who, by way of an update since last meeting, ask each other "How are you (feeling)?" However conventional it may seem, this greeting is the opening of almost all one-to-one conversations, a foreword with the implication of "first things first."

This implication has been paraphrased in Descartes' statement that "health is the chief blessing and fountain of all the other blessings in this life." Although standing in the pantheon with such other universal values as justice, truth, love and freedom, health among Western thinkers has received nothing like the continuing critical examinations that have been made of the other basic goods of life.[25]

Microbiologist René Dubos of Rockefeller University was in the vanguard of critics of medicine's prevailing, pathology-fixed tunnel vision: "Solving problems of disease is not the same thing as creating health…this task demands a kind of wisdom and vision which transcends specialized knowledge of remedies and treatments."[26] We might briefly consider this transcending proposition. In a book edited by a leading medical educator and administrator, Dr. John Knowles, we have been given a knowledgeable estimate of the relative contribution to national health of one of our largest industries, namely the practice just mentioned of "remedies and treatments." There Aaron Wildavsky writes:

> According to the Great Equation, we are told, Medical Care equals Health. But the Great Equation is wrong. More available medical care does not equal better health. The best estimates are that the medical system (doctors, drugs, hospitals) affects about 10 percent of the usual indices for measuring health: whether you live at all (infant mortality), how well you live (days lost due to sickness), how long you live

(adult mortality); the remaining 90 percent are determined by factors over which [patient care] doctors have little or no control, from individual life style, to social conditions, to the physical environment. Most of the bad things that happen to people are at present beyond the reach of medicine.[27]

Thus the 90 percent beyond the help of patient-care physicians defines the area of health left to public health professionals and their research auxiliaries, including behavioral scientists.

To be sure, clinical evidence derived from patients in treatment offers the physician intensive insights into pathologies. However it also imposes a constricted view of the broader horizon of incipient subpathologic and prepathologic levels of health not usually seen in the clinic early enough.[28] As we shall presently note, the Midtown investigation from the start measured the entire scope of health differences in its sampled community population.

Toward placing the present research within the full semantic spread of words related to health, the reader might briefly note the etymology of this key concept. Its root is "hal," the eleventh century ancestor of the modern "whole," suggesting a spectrum of deficiencies falling short of wholeness, rather than medicine's traditional either-or dichotomy of the sick and the well. The two derivative terms, "heal" and "well" are the original bases for the modern sharp distinction within the professional structure of medicine between (1) the physician's fee-for-patient-care functions in one-to-one "hands on" settings, and (2) the "public health" functions, many performed at some distance from the individual citizen by publicly supported professionals.[29] The latter seek at minimum to reduce or delay a population's need for healing; or, worded differently, to maintain increasing numbers of its people in a state of wellness, by mass education and environmental research and intervention. Metaphorically, it can be said, the latter are "crisis preventers," or "health conservers," as distinguished from their patient-care counterparts who are "crisis managers" for already sick individuals.

Of course the crisis managers apply the criteria of visible "illness" for admission to treatment, but tend to dismiss the rest of the public as being in "the gray state of health corresponding to the absence of full-blown disease."[30] The public health "conservers," on the other hand, accept responsibility for monitoring an entire community and its habitat. Systematic research monitoring, called "epidemiology," usually screens a general home-based population for one or more classes of deviations from the wholeness implied by the familiar phrases "in the best of health" or "hale and hearty."

In the Midtown studies, the class that is our primary, but by no means sole concern, is mental or emotional health. Of course this emphasis is related to the immediate contexts of sponsorship by psychiatry departments in the Cornell (MHIM1) and Columbia (MHIM2) faculties of medically-allied professions, and, as already indicated, the principal support by the National Institute of Mental Health. For a number of reasons, including the novelty and public health-policy implications of our findings, this pinpointed center has monopolized most of the MHIM1 data analysis operations and corpus of publications. However, in our sights, through both Midtown I and II, have been a series of three other types of life outcomes, outer rings on our target, their results reported together for the first time within these covers.

This is the entire series, as applied to all of our research subjects:

1. Mental/emotional health
2. Somatic health
3. Intrafamily economic well-being (socioeconomic status, or SES)
4. Extra-family social ties (social network density)

Each of these domains is seen as a ladder of differences among people classed according to how favorable or unfavorable they are to their well-being. And since each level of difference is usually derived from identical sets of information obtained both in 1954 and in 1974, one of our investigative aims is the nature of the panel's twenty-year up-and-down shifts on each of the domain-specific ladders.

To be emphasized is our view that the above domains are analytically, but not substantively, separable behavioral spheres. In reality they are seamless facets in the inclusive oneness of the functioning human being, comprehending the intrapsychic/somatic/interpersonal "trinity" commonly referred to today in medicine and public health as "biopsychosocial."[31]

We would not leave the reader with the impression that the public health orientation and biopsychosocial configuration just outlined were fully formulated in 1954. Like all Western-bred people, the study team at that time had been indelibly impressed early on with the dominant authority of the patient-care physician, and subsequently several of them, including the senior author, had ancillary roles in training medical personnel. However it is relevant to note for the record that four earlier influences were already moving to bring about the comprehensive orientation presented above. In chronological sequence they were:

1. The French sociologist, Émile Durkheim, who demonstrated that the biological human animal, pre-adult or otherwise, can survive only as a social being.[32]

2. The Swiss-American psychiatrist, Adolf Meyer, who challenged patient care specialists' fixations on this or that malfunctioning organ rather than the whole person.[33]

3. International in origin, the constitution of the World Health Organization, drafted in 1948 by public health leaders, specified as its ultimate objective for the year 2000 "the attainment by all peoples of the highest possible level of health," with "highest level" referring to "a state of complete physical, mental and social well-being, and not merely the absence of disease or infirmity."[34]

4. The Franco-American, scientist-philosopher, René Dubos, whose book *Mirage of Health* was largely a call, supported by wide medical, anthropological and historical learning, to the comprehensive perspective that "apprehends in all their complexities and subtleties the relations between living things and their total environments."[35]

From the beginning the Midtown study team were mindful of these four influences, and brought them into the Study's targeted framework. However the urgent contextual atmosphere described as enveloping the investigation from birth onward immediately narrowed the innermost circle on their target to the last words in the title of the funding Institute, namely, "mental health."

How to define and measure this elusive quality in a large population had long been a source of professional controversy. One clinical psychiatrist summarized the situation for his fellow specialists as late as 1975:

> There is no single definition of mental health that comes anywhere near to encompassing a general professional consensus...mental disease turns out to be as ill-defined as mental health. Its presence or absence is very hard to determine.[36]

However a partial operational solution to the problem had surfaced from the rival field of psychometrics, in its development of standardized, systematic symptom inventories that had been thoroughly pretested in a variety of populations. A subcommittee of the study team reviewed all the symptom questions in this series of inventories, and with Dr. Rennie as preceptor, selected 83 of these with a "current" time reference, for inclusion in its interview schedule. The sample respondent, then, reported the recent presence or absence of each covered symptom in turn.

The next challenging problem to face us was how to reliably classify this large corpus of information from each Midtown sample member. Toward a solution Dr. Rennie avoided the controversial either-or distinction between "sick" and "not sick." Instead he arranged six classes of symptom-formation clusters on a continuum according to the number and psychic severity of symptoms reported. These were labelled consecutively:

1. No significant symptoms (Well).
2. Mild array of symptoms.
3. Moderate array of symptoms.
4. Marked, life-handicapping symptoms.
5. Severe social-role crippling symptoms.
6. Incapacitating dependence on others.

When statistically imperative Rennie merged classes 4, 5, and 6 into the category of *functionally impaired mental health* (Impaired).

He trained two younger associate clinical psychiatrists in applying this schema to extracts of our respondents' interview records.[37] To be emphasized is that the associate psychiatrists each separately read the extracts from the respondents' interviews, and for each part independently assigned them to one of the six Rennie grades of symptom formation.[38]

This laborious rating procedure was necessary to test the Study's most fundamental theorem: Aspects of sociocultural contextual settings (in both their normative and deviant forms) operating both inside and outside of the family, during childhood and adulthood, have measurable consequences reflected in differences in mental health composition among subgroups within a community population.

This proposition referred to such a wide range of biopsychosocial processes that the senior social scientist for analytical purposes divided it into ten areas. Relative to adult mental health as an outcome, six were determined at birth through one's parentage, and accordingly could not be influenced by the respondent's subsequent mental health[39]. These were:

1. Age order, as defined by year of birth.
2. Gender.
3. Parental socioeconomic status.
4. Generation in the United States in three groups, immigrants, children, of immigrants, and grandchildren of immigrants and beyond.
5. Religious origin of parents in four groups, Catholic, Protestant, Jewish, and Other.

6. Nationality origin of parents in seven groups, German-Austrian, Irish, Czechoslovakian, Hungarian, Italian, British, and Puerto Rican.

The four remaining areas were largely the result of the respondents' own actions, and therefore interact with their adult mental health:

1. Marital status in four groups, never married, married, divorced-separated, and widowed.
2. Own current socioeconomic status.
3. Pre-Midtown rural-urban provenance in four groups, rural, town, middle-size city, and big city.
4. Own religious affiliation, in four groups, Catholic, Protestant, Jewish, and Other.

In some 300 pages of *Mental Health in the Metropolis*, the senior author and his colleagues studied the ranks of the above groups on the six-level yardstick of current mental health. For the detailed results of these analyses we must refer the reader to that volume.[40] Here we can share several pivotal findings with the reader.

1. In the sample as a whole a clear majority of respondents fell into the Mild and Moderate levels of symptom formation, with minorities appearing in the extreme Well and Impaired levels. The Mild level in particular had the largest representation, making it the most typical grade in the population.

2. There were remarkable similarities of proportions in the intermediate Mild and Moderate levels across the entire sample population, no matter how it was subdivided according to the ten specified sociocultural areas.

3. However statistically significant intergroup frequencies in the Well and Impaired levels were found. That is, the Mild and Moderate proportions were more or less the same among our many sociocultural groups. On the other hand, where the proportion of a group in the Well level was relatively large, the proportion in the Impaired level was relatively small, and vice versa. Graphically stated, the two levels behaved differently from each other in contrasting ways, somewhat in the manner of two children perched on opposite ends of a playground see-saw.

In the light of this pattern we devised a new measure, the group ratio of number of Impaired subjects per 100 Well subjects, called the Impaired/Well ratio. Where the total memberships of groups were sufficiently large, this elementary statistic provided a single summary.

4. The most important etiological finding of MHIM1 was this: We first ranked the Midtowners by which of the six levels of the independent variable of parental SES (during the respondent's childhood) they fell into. We then found that Midtowners raised in poverty-level families had in their ranks almost five times as many Impaired people per 100 Well as had Midtowners raised by wealthy or affluent parents (Srole et al., 1975). When grouped by the other independent variables, Generation in the United States, Religious Origin, and National Origin of Parents, Midtowners did not differ in mental health as long as their level of parental SES was controlled (i.e., held constant).

5. This finding presented MHIM2 with its major hypothesis, which can be stated in the form of two propositions:

a. Aspects of families' higher or lower positions in their community's socioeconomic structure influence both the personal life of family members within the family and their interactions with other persons outside the family; this creates drastically different settings for children to grow into and out of.

b. These differences begin to influence children's biopsychosocial development during their most impressionable, formative years.

6. Thus we postulate that, according to their SES position, parents and the family life setting within which they socialize the child play a crucial part in the development of the child's vulnerabilities and resistances to mental health risk factors throughout the entire span of the life cycle.[41]

7. We further propose that these processes may be different for children of each gender, in measurable ways. That is, the life cycle antecedents of adult mental health may be different for the Midtown women than for the Midtown men, reaching back to their early life experience and biosocial background (age, gender, and parental SES).

8. We will explore these propositions using the life-cycle data provided by the Midtowners, examining not only similarities and differences in the biopsychosocial antecedents of adult mental health but also of the health-related life-outcomes of severity of somatic disorders and affective symptom formation. These propositions first imply that aspects of the Midtowners' reported early life experiences are associated with their biosocial background characteristics. Secondly, these propositions imply that both biosocial background characteristics and early life experience are associated with health-related life outcomes in adulthood, both in 1954 and in 1974. The complexity of these propositions can be reduced by the actual statistical findings of our investi-

gations, at least in terms of the story of the lifespan development of our Midtowners' health. That is, we do not accept the fundamental theorem as a necessary truth, but rather seek to test it by analyzing the associations we observe over the life cycle of our Midtowners.[42] We further seek to define the extent to which the life cycle development of the Midtown women's health is similar to or different from that of the Midtown men.

Midtown II's (MHIM2) Research Methods

We will now briefly describe the way in which the Midtown II study of 1974 was carried out. We first established that a follow-up study could be validly done twenty years later by conducting a Trace Operation which located 1,124 of the original 1,660 Midtowners. (A full report on this state-of-the-art project follows this Introduction.) Among those located, 858 were alive and 266 were deceased. Of those found alive, 81 percent (N=695) were reinterviewed in 1974. Among the total unlocated at the close of field work (N=536), we actuarially estimated that 100 had died (mostly the oldest men and women). Among the unlocated Midtowners were 129 women who had been either unmarried or formerly married in 1954. Since they had not only relocated but very likely also acquired new surnames, by marriage or remarriage, they could not be traced.

On the basis of multiple systematic comparisons of the 695 Midtowners who were reinterviewed with the total 1954 sample of 1,660 Midtowners, we have concluded that they are equivalent in both demography and behavior. There are only several departures from this equivalence, of accurately measured and relatively small magnitude. These differences are as might be expected in a follow-up study after a twenty-year duration: the proportion in the oldest age group is lower in 1974 (19 percent) than in 1954 (27 percent); the proportion of lower SES is less in 1974 (25 percent) than in 1954 (33 percent); the proportion of higher SES is greater in 1974 (43 percent) than in 1954 (34 percent), and the proportion of younger women is less in 1974 (21 percent) than in 1954 (27 percent).

5. Whereas the 1954 interview took an average of 90 minutes to complete, the Midtowners were asked a far broader and more detailed range of questions about their somatic, psychological, and social health and well-being in 1974, so that the reinterview took an average of three hours to complete. We sought to assess their ability to deal with unfa-

vorable as well as favorable life experiences in the twenty years from 1954 to 1974.

Thus we made sure that the Midtowners would tell the whole story of how they lived through four most important portions of their life cycle, either in the 1954 or in the 1974 interviews:

a. Their early life experience, from early childhood to the end of their teen years at age 19. (This area had been intensively explored in the 1954 interview, but some needed additional data was obtained in 1974.)
b. Their baseline adult characteristics in 1954 (the Midtown I year).
c. Life cycle developments from 1954 to 1974.
d. Their terminal adult characteristics in 1974 (the Midtown II year).

The single most important part of the 1974 interview was the repetition of the 83 symptom items from the 1954 interview on which the two psychiatrists had based their ratings of the degree to which the Midtowners had functionally impaired mental health. Since these two psychiatrists were no longer available in 1974, we could not have them repeat their ratings twenty years later. However we were able to use the step-wise multiple regression analysis method to produce a statistically acceptable substitute rating, based upon a weighted composite of twenty-two items which predicted the 1954 psychiatrists' ratings discrete of each other and the remaining 61 symptom items (multiple correlation = 0.83) (Singer 1976). Each item is weighted by the degree to which it predicts the psychiatrists' ratings. These weighted items are then added. The totals are divided into six levels so that the percentage of Midtowners falling into each of the six levels is the same as the percentage which fell into each of the six levels of the psychiatrists' ratings.

In MHIM2 we use only this statistical substitute rating as our measure of adult mental health. The level of this rating based upon the Midtowners' response to the items asked in 1954 is called MH54, while the level based upon their response to the same items asked in 1974 is called MH74. The twenty-two items which were found to satisfactorily reproduce the psychiatrists' ratings were as follows[43]:

1. Did you ever have a nervous breakdown? (1=Yes, 0=No)

2. When you go out, do you usually prefer to go by yourself? (1=Yes, 2=No)

3. I am bothered by acid (sour) stomach several times a week. (1=Yes, 2=No)

4. Are you ever bothered by nervousness? (1=Often, 2=Sometimes, 3=Never)

5. Do you sometimes feel that people are against you without any good reason? (1=Yes, 2=No)

6. Interviewer rating: R's tension level at start. (1=Nervous, 2=Sporadic Nervousness, 3=Mostly Relaxed)

7. Behind your back, people say all kinds of things about you. (1=Disagree, 2=Agree)

8. I have had periods of weeks or months when I couldn't take care of things because I couldn't get going. (1=Yes, 2=No)

9. Feelings of grief and sorrow are suitable for children but not for adults. (1=Disagree, 2=Agree)

10. I often have a hard time making up my mind about things I should do. (1=Yes, 2=No)

11. Like a lot of people, do you sometimes drink more than is good for you? (1=Yes, 0=No)

12. Have you ever had a fainting spell? (1=Never, 2=A few times, 3=More than a few times)

13. About your health[44] now, would you say it is excellent, good, fair, or poor? (1=Excellent, 2=Good, 3=Fair, 4=Poor)

14. I have periods of such great restlessness that I cannot sit long in a chair. (1=Yes, 2=No)

15. To avoid arguments, do you usually keep your opinions to yourself? (1=Yes, 2=No)

16. I have personal worries that get me down physically. (1=Disagree, 2=Agree)

17. Do you ever have any trouble in getting to sleep? (1=Often, 2=Sometimes, 3=Never)

18. Certain kinds of places make me tense such as high buildings, tunnels, or bridges. (1=Disagree, 2=Agree)

19. Do you feel somewhat apart, even among friends? (1=Yes, 2=No)

20. Have you ever been bothered by shortness of breath when you were not exercising or working hard? (1=Often, 2=Sometimes, 3=Never)

21. How often are you worried by loneliness? (1=Often, 2=Sometimes, 3=Never)

22. Have you ever had spells of dizziness? (1=Never, 2=A few times, 3=More than a few times)

MHIM2's Principal Findings

This book is devoted to presenting the principal findings of MHIM2 with respect to mental health and its primary associated biopsychosocial correlates. While we must leave the intricate details to the body of the book, overall this is what we have found:

1. The average level of mental health remains the same over the twenty-year period. Thus there are no detectible subsequent cumulative impacts of the period 1954 to 1974 on the Midtowners' mental health. In fact a smaller proportion of these reinterviewed Midtowners are Impaired in 1974 than in 1954, and a greater proportion are Well in 1974 than in 1954, but their preponderance in the Mild and Moderate levels of mental health keeps the average level the same.

2. We next examine the extent to which Midtowners' membership in an "earlier" or "later" generation (as defined as whether they were of age 40–59 in 1954 versus in 1974) is associated with their level of mental health.[45] We find that there is a difference between the two generations of Midtown women, but not between the two generations of Midtown men. A larger proportion of earlier Midtown women had impaired mental health as compared with later Midtown women. In contrast, the two generations of Midtown men had equal average levels of mental health; and about equal proportions of Midtown earlier and later men had either well or impaired mental health.

Thus the MH of the Midtown women changed between two historical generations in a manner not paralleled by the stability of their MH over twenty years of biosocial aging. In contrast the MH of the Midtown men did not change either over two historical generations or over twenty years of biosocial aging. The facts that there was no change in adult mental health observed after twenty years of biosocial aging and that a difference in adult mental health at age 40–59 between two historical generations is observed only among the Midtown women suggest the extent to which adult mental health is rooted in the preadult years.

3. We have been quite intrigued by the fact that the two generations of Midtown women differ in their mental health composition at age 40–59 whereas the two generations of Midtown men did not so differ. To attempt to further understand this finding in the context of our data on the whole life cycle, we use multiple regression (or path) analysis to determine the extent to which four types of biopsychosocial antecedents of adult mental health might differently predict the mental health level of the Midtown earlier and later men and women. These types of biopsychosocial antecedents are:

a. *Biosocial Background*: Age, Gender, and Parental SES.

b. *Contexts of Childhood Functioning*: Body Damage (the degree of whole-ness of physical constitution starting from early childhood), Parental Intrafamily Functioning, Parental Breadwinner Adequacy, and Family-Kin Network.

c. *Pre-Adult Well-Being*: A combination of measures of the Midtowners' pre-adult physical health, mental health, and social well-being.

d. *Severity of Somatic Disorders Up To 1954*: Each physical health disorder which Midtowners report in 1974 that they had had by 1954 is weighted by the physician-rated seriousness of that disorder. All of these weights are then summed. Midtowners might score high on this measure either by having had a few physical health disorders rated by physicians as being relatively serious, or by having had many physical health disorders rated by physicians as being relatively mild or moderate in seriousness.

We find that parental SES is associated with the pre-adult well-being and adult mental health of the earlier Midtown women in a way that it is not in either the later Midtown women or in either the earlier or later Midtown men: Among the earlier Midtown women, parental SES predicts their level of pre-adult well-being, which in turn predicts their level of 1954 adult mental health. When the prediction of their MH54 by their level of parental SES is adjusted for their level of pre-adult well-being, it is reduced to virtually zero. Thus among the earlier Midtown women, disadvantageous parental SES set the stage for less favorable than average pre-adult well-being, which in turn led to less favorable than average adult mental health. But among the remaining Midtowners, there is in fact no correlation between parental SES and pre-adult well-being, that is, among the later Midtown women and the Midtown men of both generations, disadvantageous parental SES does *not* set the stage for less favorable than average pre-adult well-being. Yet among both the earlier and later Midtown men and women, pre-adult well-being significantly predicts adult mental health at age 40–59. Thus the *childhood* functioning of the earlier Midtown women who came from socioeconomically disadvantaged families appears to have been uniquely adversely impacted whereas the childhood functioning of the later Midtown women and of the earlier and later Midtown men from socioeconomically disadvantaged families was not adversely impacted. And overall the best predictor of MH54 is childhood functioning (pre-adult well-being).

4. We have also explored in similar fashion the life cycle bio-psychosocial antecedents of the adult mental health of our Midtowners in 1954 and in 1974. We have paid particular attention to possible differences in how our biopsychosocial life-span model might differ-

ently predict the adult mental health of the Midtown women vis-à-vis the Midtown men. We have also explored the distribution and antecedents of a number of important biopsychosocial correlates of adult mental health in a way paralleling our investigation of MH.

We note that the field of gender specificity in life course is understandably confusing to those who have studied it in the past twenty years. Depending upon which aspects one might investigate, women and men might appear to have their lives influenced by very similar factors in parallel ways, similar factors but in divergent ways, completely different factors, or some combination. We conclude that to understand an aspect of the life course, both genders must be studied as much in the same way as possible, that is, sampled and measured the same way: for after reviewing all of the analyses on which this monograph is based, we found that, (excluding the predictions of Gender and Gender by Age Level), of 201 statistically significant predictions made by our biographical model, about half or 93 (46.3 percent) are cross-gender, about a third or 65 (32.3 percent) are probably specific to the Midtown women, and about a fifth or 43 (21.4 percent) are probably specific to the Midtown men. The Midtown women are somewhat more likely to have the aspects of their life span studied in this monograph predicted by factors specific to them than are the Midtown men, as the predictions are distributed among the three types (cross-gender, probably specific to the women, and probably specific to the Men) in a ratio of 5:3:2.[46]

* * *

Having summarized in a general way the findings of MHIM2 we turn now to a discussion of the state-of-the-art trace operation which made the restudy possible.

Notes

1. That is, the present senior author and his colleagues of 1954.
2. (a) Srole, Langner et al. 1962; (b) Srole, Langer et al. 1975; (c) Srole, Langer et al. 1978.
3. In one noteworthy instance, the correspondence had an unbroken duration of thirty-four years.
4. This kind of personal change has since been intimated by investigative journalist J. Anthony Lucas in his 1985 best-seller, a meticulous documentation of ten years of racial crisis in inner-city Boston. Lucas there writes, inter alia, that he was "drawn" to the "families at the center of my story by [their] engagement with life, which made them stand out from their social context...The realities of urban America, when seen through the lives of actual city dwellers, proved far more complicated than I had imagined."

5. Lidz 1968; Offer and Sabshin 1984.
6. Stevenson 1966: vii–viii.
7. Simonton 1990.
8. It seems to be an uncanny coincidence that the Academy of Motion Pictures Award-winning foreign language film *A Man and A Woman*, released in 1965, has been followed by a sequel entitled *A Man and A Woman: Twenty Years Later*, with the same author-director and the same characters played by the same actors. With his characters now in their mid-fifties the film's director, Claude Lelouch, observed that "theirs is the beautiful age for a love story. The seat of power rests with people of that age, and kids of twenty-five are more old-fashioned than their parents." *New York Times*, 11 October 1985. On another level, the film is viewed by a Hollywood director, Sydney Pollack, as "a way to examine what's happened to you over the years (ibid.)."
9. Of course, the Study Director's original guarantee of confidentiality of the subject's personal identity and information continues inviolate.
10. A more recent manifestation of this ongoing situation is revealing. A huge new "luxury" housing development has been built on the most northern block in the Midtown area, with guest entrances at its southern (95th Street) face, and "service" entrances at its northern (96th Street) face.
11. Among the better known are Carnegie Hill, Gracie Square, Lenox Hill, and Yorkville.
12. To this day, taxi drivers of the five counties and the *U.S. Postal Zip Code Directory* confuse newcomers and tourists by continuing to refer to Manhattan as the "City of New York."
13. The original designation of "Greater New York" has long been dropped from popular use, except by political and Chamber of Commerce officials, to refer to the more inclusive metropolitan region.
14. Kessler and Levin, eds. 1970.
15. For details see Srole, Langner et al. 1962.
16. The pros and cons of that sort of study were subsequently explored in Cedric X (1973: 1–118).
17. Parker and Kleiner 1966.
18. Eli Ginzberg, et al. (NY: Columbia University Press, 1959).
19. Although on leave in late 1942 as a college professor of sociology and anthropology, the senior author was somehow classified by the United States Army Air Force for a slot as a "military psychologist," before long assigned as group therapist on a convalescent hospital ward for aircrew "psychiatric casualties." He thus became a cog in the huge system that was to be definitively analyzed a decade later by Ginzberg and his associates, under the impetus of General Eisenhower.
20. Ginzberg, pp. 58–59.
21. Faris and Dunham 1939.
22. The Psychiatric Director of the Joint Commission on Mental Illness and Health had urged that "to attain a true concept of the national [mental health] problem we need studies…of as many individual communities as possible…to be able to make comparisons between geographic, socioeconomic and cultural areas of the country." (Ewalt 1959: 622)
23. Later they were defined as seeking to order, interweave, and explain the huge array of normative and deviant human actions and reactions in their everyday social settings.
24. By sampling, "information can be drawn at relatively low cost from large populations or social universes," comparable to the "development of the telescope" (Boulding 1964: 70–71).

25. Parenthetically, at least partly responsible for this conceptual lag has been the phenomenal power-wielding ascendancy of medicine as a techno-scientifically based art (and institution), with a proprietary claim to primacy in the semantics of health. See Starr (1983: 16–21) and Illich (1976).
26. Dubos 1959: 26.
27. Wildavsky 1977: 105.
28. Among these are the "silent" coronary and cerebral infarcts and first-stage cancers of the pancreas.
29. These professionals have been represented by the American Public Health Association since 1872.
30. The matter has been paraphrased by Barbara B. Brown (1984: 2): "Between health and illness there are obscure and ambiguous states of unwellness...These states are not 'official' medical or psychological ailments. They are, instead, afflictions abandoned by the healing arts when they decided that you cannot officially feel not-well unless you are certified sick."
31. Complimentary perspectives are offered in the following references: Engel (1980: 535–544), Schwartz and Wiggins (1986: 1213–21), Antonovsky (1982), Newton et al. (1984: 230–88), and Rutter (1986: 1077–87).
32. This was dramatized in the television documentary film "Our Man in Moscow." A Russian working for British Intelligence apprehended by the Soviets is sentenced not to death but to solitary confinement, with a public announcement, however, of his execution. While his life is spared, his significant others believed he was dead. The "sociological death sentence" was so intolerable that at the first opportunity the Russian committed suicide.
33. "If science does not see that the time has come to recognize as its central concern the whole of man, as individual and group, it fails to do justice to its greatest task and opportunity" (Meyer 1935: 33).
34. Implicit here are multiple levels on a best-to-worst continuum of health.
35. Dubos 1959: 256.
36. Zusman (1975: 2327–28). Of course the introduction of DSM-III (American Psychiatric Association, 1980) brought about a uniformity in the definition of at least certain mental disorders which would have been impossible to imagine in 1954.
37. The extract was in two parts: part A—The symptomatic information; and part B—The symptomatic information plus their reported sociocultural characteristics. The rationale for this painstaking procedure is explained in the section entitled "Judgmental Bias in Psychiatric Classification," within the 1978 edition of *Mental Health in the Metropolis*, pp. 161–65. Because our associate psychiatrists' classifications based on the part B data were a closer approximation to the conventional judgmental operations of psychiatrists in their clinical practice, Dr. Rennie subsequently chose the results of the Class B 1954 classifications to be reported in all MHIM1 publications. However, for computer-driven statistical-analytic reasons discussed below, the MHIM2 results have had to be based only on the replicated Part A symptomatic information of 1974, and have been so reported in all our publications since.
38. For all sample individuals assigned differently by our two associate psychiatrists, the disagreements were systematically adjudicated with Dr. Rennie. The historical development of the mental health measure is presented in Srole (1975: 347–64). This measure has persisted in a somewhat altered form as Axis V in DSM-IV (American Psychiatric Association, 1994). An argument that it selects persons in the community as in need of psychiatric treatment more sensitively than do specific criteria for individual psychopathological syndromes is presented in Vaillant and Schnurr (1988: 313–19).

39. MHIM1 was the first cross-sectional investigation in psychiatric epidemiology to make a sharp distinction between two sets of situational-experiential factors contributing to mental health:
    a. The independent, antecedent variables, defined by the criterion that each could potentially influence the course of individual mental health development, but could hardly have been influenced by it in return. Examples are age, sex, and parental socioeconomic status, which largely defined the Midtowners' place in the social space of their childhood, one that was beyond their power to alter.
    b. The reciprocal social variables, defined by the criterion that each can be influenced by the individual's mental health, as well as potentially contribute to it. Examples are marital status and the adult's self-acquired socioeconomic status (Fischer et al., op cit.).
40. Srole et al. 1962.
41. Fischer et al., 1979. In mental health diagnostic assessment and treatment planning, these are often referred to as assets and liabilities, or strengths and weaknesses.
42. Here is a recent rejection of the biopsychosocial model in psychiatry as "revealed truth": "The multifactorial or biopsychosocial approach can be considered an improvement only if future research demonstrates that it results in an improvement in both our clinical behavior and our patients' therapeutic outcomes. One of the problems with the multifactorial approach is the difficulty created for treatment planning when etiological priority is not established" (Guscott and Grof 1991: 695–704).
43. Srole and Fischer 1980: 209–21; Srole and Fischer (1989: 35–44).
44. In 1974 this item is worded "general physical health" rather than "health."
45. Wyler et al. 1968: 363–74; 1970: 49–64.
46. See chapter 9 for a summation of our findings for mental health.

References

American Psychiatric Association. 1980. *Diagnostic and Statistical Manual of Mental Disorders*, 3d ed. Washington, DC: American Psychiatric Association.
———. 1994. *Diagnostic and Statistical Manual of Mental Disorders*, 4th ed. Washington, DC: American Psychiatric Association.
Antonovsky, Aaron. 1982. *Health, Stress, and Coping*. San Francisco: Jossey-Bass Publishers.
Boulding, Kenneth E. 1964. *The Meaning of the Twentieth Century*. New York: Harper and Row.
Brown, Barbara B. 1984. *Between Health and Illness*. Princeton, NJ: Houghton Mifflin.
Dubos, René. 1959. *Mirage of Health*. New York: Harper and Row.
Engel, George L. "The clinical application of the biopsychosocial model," *American Journal of Psychiatry* 137 (May 1980): 535–44.
Ewalt, John R. "A Case for the Community Self Survey," *Public Health Reports U.S.* (July 1959): 622.
Faris, Robert E. and J. Warren Dunham. 1939. *Mental Disorders in Urban Areas*. Chicago: University of Chicago Press.
Fischer, Anita K., Janos Marton, Ernest J. Millman, and Leo Srole. 1979. "Long-range influences on adult mental health: The Midtown Manhattan Longitudinal Study, 1954–1974," in *Research in Community and Mental Health, Vol. 1*, edited by Roberta G. Simmons, 305–33. Greenwich, CT: JAI Press.

Guscott, Richard and Paul Grof. "The Clinical Meaning of Refractory Depression: A Review for the Clinician." *American Journal of Psychiatry* 148 (June 1991): 695–704.

Illich, Ivan. 1976. *Medical Nemesis: The Expropriation of Health.* New York: Panetheon Books, Random House.

Kessler, Irving I. and Morton I. Levin, eds. 1970. *The Community As an Epidemiologic Laboratory.* Baltimore, MD: Johns Hopkins Press.

Lidz, Theodore. 1968. *The Person.* New York: Basic Books.

Lucas, J. Anthony. 1985. *Common Ground.* New York: A.A. Knopf.

Meyer, Adolf. "The Birth and Development of the Mental-Hygiene Movement." *Mental Hygiene* 19 (January 1935): 29–36.

Newton, Nancy A., Lawrence W. Lazarus, and Jack Weinberg. 1984. "Aging: biopsychosocial perspectives". In *Normality and the Life Cycle: A Critical Integration,* edited by Daniel Offer and Melvin Sabshin, 230–88. New York: Basic Books.

Parker, Seymour and Robert J. Kleiner. 1966. *Mental Illness in the Urban Negro Community.* New York: The Free Press.

Rutter, Michael. "Meyerian psychobiology, personality development, and the role of life experiences." *American Journal of Psychiatry* 143 (September 1986): 1077–87.

Schwartz, Michael A. and Osborne P. Wiggins. "Systems and the structuring of meaning: contributions to a biopsychosocial medicine." *American Journal of Psychiatry* (October 1986): 1213–21.

Simonton, Dean K. 1990. *Psychology, Science, and History: An Introduction to Historiometry.* New Haven, CT: Yale University.

Singer, Eleanor, Steven M. Cohen, Robin Garfinkel, and Leo Srole. "Replicating psychiatric ratings through multiple regression analysis: The Midtown Manhattan Restudy." *Journal of Health and Social Behavior* 17 (December 1976): 376–87.

Srole, Leo. "Measurement and classification in sociopsychiatric epidemiology: The Midtown Manhattan Study (1954) and Midtown Manhattan Restudy (1974)," *Journal of Health and Social Behavior* 16 (December 1975): 347–64.

Srole, Leo and Anita K. Fischer. *Changing lives and well-being: the Midtown Manhattan Panel Study, 1954–1976* (sic). *Acta Psychiatrica Scandanavia* 79 (suppl. 348, 1989): 35–44.

———. "The Midtown Manhattan Longitudinal Study vs. 'The Mental Paradise Lost' doctrine: a controversy joined." *Archives of General Psychiatry* 37 (February 1980): 209–21.

Srole, Leo, Thomas S. Langner, Marvin K. Opler, and Thomas A. C. Rennie. 1962. *Mental Health in the Metropolis, Vol. 1 of the Midtown Manhattan Study.* New York: Blakiston Division, McGraw-Hill.

Srole, Leo, Thomas S. Langner, Stanley T. Michael, Price Kirkpatrick, Marvin K. Opler, and Thomas A. C. Rennie. 1975. *Mental Health in the Metropolis: The Midtown Manhattan Study.* Enlarged and revised edition, edited by Leo Srole and Anita K. Fischer. New York: Harper and Row Torchbooks.

———. 1978. *Mental Health in the Metropolis: The Midtown Manhattan Study.* Revised and enlarged edition. Edited by Leo Srole and Anita K. Fischer. New York: New York University Press.

Starr, Paul. 1983. *The Social Transformation of American Medicine.* New York: Basic Books.

Stevenson, Earl P. 1986. "Foreword," in *Social Indicators,* edited by Raymond A. Bauer, vii–viii. Cambridge, MA: M.I.T. Press.

Vaillant, George, and Paula Schnurr. "What is a case? A 45-year study of psychiatric impairment of a college sample selected for mental health." *Archives of General Psychiatry* 45 (April 1988): 313–19.

Wildavsky, Aaron. 1977. "Doing Better, Feeling Worse: The Political Pathology of Health Policy," in *Doing Better and Feeling Worse: Health in the United States,* edited by John H. Knowles, 105–24. New York: W. W. Norton.

Wyler, Allen R., Minoru Masuda, and Thomas H. Holmes. "The Seriousness of Illness rating scale." *Journal of Psychosomatic Research* 11 (December 1968): 363–74.

Wyler, Allen R., Minoru Masuda, and Thomas H. Holmes. "The Seriousness of Illness rating scale: reproducibility." *Journal of Psychosomatic Research* 14 (March 1970): 49–64.

Cedric X (Clark) ed., "The White Researcher in Black Society," special issue of *The Journal of Social Issues,* 29 (Winter 1973): 1–118.

Zusman, Jack. 1975. "Primary Prevention," in *Comprehensive Textbook in Psychiatry II,* vol. 2, edited by Alexander M. Freedman, Harold I. Kaplan, and Benjamin J. Sadock, 2327–28. Baltimore, MD: Williams and Wilkins.

2

Midtowners Lost and Found:
Search and Assessment—Tactics and Results[1]

How Representative are the Midtown II Reinterviewees?

One of the first of the general population public health investigations ever fielded, the original Midtown Study had to improvise its way through a newly opened research frontier. From total immersion in the "here and now" of an untrodden stand of metaphorical trees, we did not envision the forest's enlarged scientific significance a generation later. Myopic short-sightedness beset the young behavioral sciences of the period.

Followup of our 1660 Midtowners came as an afterthought, an opportunity to net for another few hours those early "birds on the wing"—and only those—an enterprise equivalent to a naturalist's subsequent return to the bird's individual nesting places, new or otherwise. To revisit a large roster of specific individual householders after a substantial passage of time requires careful pre-planning. In the absence of 20/20 foresight, the Midtown interview schedule of 1954 did not ask for the particular kinds of personal linkages, beyond household fellow-occupants (if any[2]), who could help retrace the steps leading to our subjects' subsequent dwelling habitats.

Years later, as we began to consider Midtown II, we confronted the uncertainty of retrieving a Midtown I subsample ("panel")[3] of sufficiently large numbers to serve as a representative surrogate of the original sample. To resolve this uncertainty, our proposal to conduct a feasibility test was accorded sponsorship by Professor Lawrence C. Kolb, chairman of the Columbia Department of Psychiatry, with encouragement by National Institute of Mental Health professional staff and approval by the Institute's review and advisory bodies.[4]

With such strong backing, we mobilized our all-out Trace Operation, targeting each of our original 1660 subjects, without any exclusions whatsoever[5], applying the identical battery of search techniques toward giving all the same chance of leading us to their whereabouts, even to the last home address of those deceased.[6]

The closest hypothetical approximation to the Operation's mandate would have been that of a small team of investigative journalists seeking to locate (and interview) a large aggregate of people last contacted several decades earlier, but now in possession of critical new information only they could provide.

After the obvious "first pass" approaches through "Please Forward" letters, telephone "Information" requests and relevant organization directories, we began address searches through face-to-face "networking" inquiries of ex-neighbors, building superintendents, local shopkeepers, real estate agents, etc., then combed the often inadequate (pre-computerized) public records of various federal, state and city institutions, including, for example, hospitals, social services, welfare offices, motor vehicle bureaus, and the inpatient archives of the New York State Department of Mental Health. Our "trace histories" on all missing subjects themselves required a bookkeeping register of our own to record "bases touched," and to follow new leads for further tracking.

At the end of this comprehensive sweep, all Midtown I subjects fell into one of three inclusive categories: (1) the "reported" deceased; (2) the "tentative" unlocated; and (3) the located alive. Names in the first category usually began as word-of-mouth reports that we systematically checked against New York State death certificates for verifying information to match items in our 1954 interview records.[7]

As an independent test of the exhaustiveness of our trace efforts with the unlocated category, we selected twenty of their number who seemed to offer the most promising prospects for tracking by field personnel of the Pinkerton Detective Agency, working from their own resources and the best information already in our possession. Their "found" rate was identical with our own—zero.

The Pinkerton report was an "end-of-the-line" signal to the search phase of Operation Trace; remaining was the follow-through phase of assessing its results. Toting up "the bottom line," we had now verified the whereabouts of 1124 subjects, or 67.7 percent of our entire Midtown I sample: 858 of them alive, 266 deceased, and 536 (32.8 percent) "terminally" unlocatable.

Operation Trace: Assessment Phase

The Located Alive were felt to be a numerically feasible subsample for a reinterview study. However the large total of Unlocateds posed an inescapable challenge. If the Pinkerton agent is powerless to retrieve the terminally unlocatable, the scientist who commissioned him has the option (1) to "close the books" on them, or (2) to take a further step, namely, to sort them into several explanatory types from available Midtown I information. We took that step in order to identify the subgroup sources of those "lost to follow-up," and to assess the consequences of their absence for the significance of the larger Located Alive aggregate remaining within reach.

If the search phase had required the familiar "shoe leather" methods of investigative journalists, the assessment phase demanded the classical deductive methods of the detective craft in ferreting key unknowns out of the knowns in hand.

The reader may wish to follow our own analytic deductive efforts to identify different categories among the Unlocateds of 1974. We began by sorting them according to their gender and marital status in 1954. This quickly led to the discovery of an excess number of never-marrieds (NM) among the unlocated females. Similarly, focusing on the Located Alive of 1974, we found that the NM of 1954 showed up twenty years later with contrasting proportions of the sexes who, in the interval, had married, namely 60 percent of the men and only 25 percent of the women, an unusually large discrepancy. However we could surmise a connection between (1) this unexpected deficit of the NM women of 1954 in the Located Alive of 1974, and (2) the 1974 excess of unlocated women who, in 1954, had been unmarried.

The deduced link followed from this known: unlike their male counterparts, women upon marriage as a rule move to another address and drop their maiden surname for their husband's, in effect substituting a culturally contrived alias. Inevitably, the combined change of both residence and surname confounds further trace efforts[8] with predictable results.

Taking all available clues into account, we could conservatively estimate that some 110 of the 256 NM females of 1954 (documented then as a predominantly young, employed and healthy subgroup) were diverted by an intervening cultural barrier from our Located Alive category, posing a question as to the consequences for gender differences in the reinterviewed panel that will be considered presently.

The second category under the Unlocateds arose from the certainty that hidden among them was an appreciable number of unreported (or unverifiable) cases of out-of-state deaths—but how many? To arrive at an approximate answer, we started with two knowns already elicited by Operation Trace: among the sample's total of 510 located men, the verified mortality rate had been 29.4 percent. Projecting that known mortality experience to the 180 Unlocated males, we arrived at an estimate of 53 decedents among them, or 7.7 percent of the 1954 sample total of 690 men.

Because females are known to have a lower mortality rate than their male peers, we had to modify our estimation procedure somewhat. Among the Unlocateds were a total of 246 women, exclusive of the estimated 110 ex-unmarried. We knew that the total of Located women, alive and verified dead, had a confirmed mortality frequency of 18.9 percent.

Extrapolating that rate to the 246 Unlocated females just mentioned gave us an estimated 47 of them as unreported-unverified deceased, the two sexes totalling a round 100.

The third category of Unlocateds emerges from the underclass of "outcasts"—the institutionalized and the homeless. Of the latter, in particular, the *New York Times* (30 January 1984) has written: "[they occupy] a world far outside the city that can seem—and, in fact, can be—almost impenetrable to those on the other side." (Of course similar words are more or less applicable to the long-term institutionalized.)

An illustrative case was a middle-aged unmarried female subject of upper class parentage, whom we traced to a welfare SRO hotel.[9] Repeated personal phone and written messages brought no response, until her supervising social worker reported: "She just disappeared with part of her belongings—not even her kin knew where to." On intuitive grounds we could estimate that these lost post-1954 outcasts perhaps approximated the 1.4 percent of our original sample whom we did locate and reinterview in nursing homes.

The final, heterogeneous category of Unlocateds we designate the "Residuals," who, by numerical subtraction, account for the remaining 18 percent of the total Midtown I sample. Of course, we do not know the individual reasons for their disappearance, but we can surmise that in the main they were early, and probably multiple, movers, double divorcees, job changers, and retirees, who after a succession of addresses,[10] confront the tracers with a "cold trail," in a frequency that tends to grow with them. In a finding unexpectedly opened in table 2.4 below (and there discussed), these include a discernible flow of elderly foreign-born people who have returned to their native homelands.

Could our followup have been made after an interval of ten years, let us say, our Unlocated rate would certainly have been far smaller. On the other hand, the trade-off with our opportune twenty-year interval is analogous to the gain of a time-lapse camera allowed to run at 2x, rather than 1x: More barely perceptible alterations accumulate, permitting clearer discernment of incremental changes, their differential velocities and directions becoming more reliably measurable. Needless to say, the dynamics of individual-cum-group shifts, in the face of resistance to change, is the risk-laden, potential prize attainable only with the turning of the years, as caught in the frame of long-term followup research.[11]

Addressing this point, it has been observed: "The followup is the great exposer of truth, the rocks on which fine theories are wrecked and upon which better ones can be built."[12] The general appreciation calls for the qualification that it all depends upon the time span covered. Clearly there is a considerable difference in the changes detectable as between followup of individuals from age 20 to age 22, and of the sample people from age 20 to 40.

Of course, the price, in our total Residual Unlocated rate of 18 percent (annual average 0.9 percent) is high. (The significance of its effects for the Midtown II Panel is a separate issue and remains to be explored below.) To private and public "Missing Persons Bureaus," however, an average annual 0.9 percent residual loss rate, over twenty years, would hardly seem a surprise.

Somewhat of a surprise to the reader, perhaps, is an article in *Barron's Weekly* (8 October 1984) on the sheer number of "folks who have dropped off the face of the earth," leaving behind "abandoned bank accounts, stocks and dividend checks, utility deposits and even pay checks." Such unclaimed properties, after legally mandated professional searches for their holders, ultimately revert to state treasuries, which in "the last fiscal year reaped something like $400 million" from them.

Unmentioned in the article is that largely unrepresented among this propertied "skip out" element are people at the other end of the socio-economic scale, in uncounted numbers, who, to escape creditors and abandon families, end up in the post office "Dead Letter" pigeon-hole marked "Address Unknown." In counted numbers are the two million children, nationwide, reported as missing in 1983. The overall number of "lost souls" has reached the magnitude of a national problem. This was recognized (1986) in a major television network's special series of hour-long programs devoted to actual case histories of unaccountably vanished individuals.

We might pause now to compare our average annual Residual Unlocated rate with that of several other longitudinal investigations.

The tracing problems vary enormously among them, none more so, perhaps than those confronting Midtown II. Nonetheless our annual rate (0.9 percent), although far from the lowest, is by no means the highest.[13]

Unlocatability is only the first of two major sample retrieval problems confronting longitudinal investigations. The other emerges among those located who elude reinterview by declining to participate, or are otherwise inaccessible, for reasons of distance or disability[14]; these are labelled "non-respondents," their frequency expressed in a "non-response" rate. Of course this is a problem indigenous to all sample surveys, longitudinal and otherwise.

We can now report that of the 858 original Midtowners whom we located alive, 695 were reinterviewed (including 13 of the 18 living in Canada, Europe, Africa, or Asia) and 163, or 19 percent, were not. The latter figure is somewhat larger than the 13 percent non-response in our younger, designated sample of 1954. In the decades that followed, however, sample surveys generally have reported accelerating increases in this rate. A typical example is presented in a replicated, large-scale national mental health survey conducted in 1976 by the respected Survey Research Center of the University of Michigan. The authors report that 29 percent of their designated sample were not interviewed, a frequency they consider "a serious problem" and elaborate: "When non-response rates get over 20 or 25 percent, the representativeness of the [interviewed] sample must be questioned...Non-responses have been found most frequently in densely populated metropolitan centers. [The SRC] non-response rate for New York City in 1976 was 40 percent."[15] This frequency is twice larger than our own at about the same time, in more or less the same region.

Detecting Subsample Bias of Genders
Culled from the Midtown I Sample

Given unlocatability and non-response among the located, long-term followup studies are open to the hazard of ending with a reinterviewed panel that is demographically biased—in the sense that it may overrepresent population groups easy to retrieve, and underrepresent groups equally (or more) important, but difficult to corral. If so, its representative significance may be impaired, when the overriding of a sample is to yield and project valid conclusions to a larger specific population universe of major scientific interests.

TABLE 2.1
Distribution of Terminal Trace and Reinterview
Categories in Midtown I Sample by Genders

	Men (N = 690)	Women (N = 970)
I. Located Dead (verified)	21.9%	11.9%
II. Unlocated (estimated)		
A. Ex non-married women	—	11.3%
B. Deceased	7.7%	4.8%
C. In institutions, homeless	0.7%	1.0%
D. Residual	17.4%	19.7%
Subtotal	47.7%	48.7%
III. Located Alive		
A. Reinterviewed (The "Panel")	42.6%	41.3%
B. Not Reinterviewed	9.7%	10.0%
Subtotal	52.3%	51.3%

To settle this overhanging uncertainty, we are inviting the reader to share our surgical excursions into the Midtown I sample's demographic innards for major imbalances, witting or otherwise.

The genders are a pair of groups especially vulnerable to unequal chances of inclusion during sample recruitment.[16] To explore this particular possibility, table 2.1 is the first of our accountings promised above. It records the gender-specific 1974 distributions on the Terminal Trace and reinterview categories that were extracted from the entire Midtown sample of 1954.

Turning to that table, we note the "Bias of Survival," whereby more women tend to survive than do men of like age, and the "Bias of Matrimony" in Western culture, whereby only women at marriage change their patronym (for their husband's).[17]

The residual of the above biases are evident in the differential gender rates presented in the first three rows of the table. However in the remaining five rows the pairs of gender rates are quite similar. Thus, although the total twenty-year loss to followup was considerable, our stringent operating principles and efforts brought in a panel with almost identical male and female "located alive," "reinterviewed" and "non-reinterviewed" rates.

Midtown II Panel and Located Alive Group
Compared by 1974 Areas of Residence

Table 2.1 has accounted for the results of putting the entire Midtown I sample through our screen of Trace Categories for balanced/unbalanced representations of its vulnerable gender groups. As the next step in this assessment phase, we must narrow our focus to the Midtown II Reinterviewed Panel alone, in order to compare it with a larger, partially related, population, on appropriate, known compositional characteristics. For example, we do not know the whereabouts of the Midtown I Unlocateds, but we do know the current addresses of all those located alive. Table 2.2 makes it possible to use the areas of residence of the latter entity as a yardstick to measure whether the Midtown II Reinterviewed Panel in composition is representative of the inclusive Located Alive company.[18]

Table 2.2 shows the Reinterviewed Panel's post-1954 dispersion from its original concentrated geographical base and demonstrates its close concordance with that of the entire Located Alive group. Stated differently, the non-respondents in that group impose no sampling bias, in this specific sense: Had they *all* been reinterviewed, the Panel's geographic composition would not have been significantly different from the distribution observed in the table's left-hand column.

In passing we also note that 84 percent of the Located Alive is spread across the larger metropolitan region, in concentric circles within 100

TABLE 2.2
Areas of Residential Distribution in 1974 Among Midtown II
Panel and Located Alive Group

1974 Residence	Panel (N = 695)	Located Alive (N = 858)
Same Address	20.4%	20.3%
Manhattan Other[1]	23.9%	25.4%
NYC Other	17.4%	18.4%
Counties within 50 mi. of NYC	16.4%	16.0%
Counties within 50–100 miles of NYC	5.0%	4.3%
Rest of U.S.	15.0%	13.5%
Other Countries	1.9%	2.1%
Total	100.0%	100.0%

[1] Of panelists who left Manhattan after 1954, some 7 percent by 1974 had made the round-trip back.

TABLE 2.3
Distributions on Five Sets of Major Demographic
Attributes of the Midtown II Panel in 1954

I.	Gender	
	A. Male	42.3%
	B. Female	57.7%
II.	Age	
	A. 20–29	24.0%
	B. 30–39	28.1%
	C. 40–49	28.6%
	D. 50–59	19.3%
III.	SES Background[1]	
	F. Lower Lower	11.5%
	E. Upper Lower	13.8%
	D. Lower Middle	22.6%
	C. Upper Middle	18.0%
	B. Lower Upper	15.7%
	A. Upper Upper	18.4%
IV.	Generation-in-U.S.	
	A. Foreign-born (F-B)	28.3%
	B. Children of F-B	37.8%
	C. Grandchildren	17.5%
	D. Great-grandchildren	16.4%
V.	Years of Schooling	
	A. 0–8	22.6%
	B. 9–12	40.1%
	C. 13–16	23.3%
	D. 17 or more	14.0%

[1] Based on scoring and summing of father's (a) level of education and (b) mid-life occupation.

miles of Manhattan at its core.[19] This exodus—to places as small as rural—was in part generated by processes within and around the Midtown area. In larger perspective, however, it was also a concurrent part of a much larger phenomenon, namely, a conspicuous national fanning out of inner-city white families to surrounding suburbs and exurbs. This stream was of such magnitude that by 1970, for the first time in American history, suburbanites outnumbered city dwellers (with continuing political repercussions). For evidence at levels closest to Midtown, we can estimate from Census Bureau data that between 1954 and 1974 Manhattan lost approximately 22 percent of its population, mostly whites, whereas the counties encircling the city limits swelled by about 25 percent.

Close-up of Panel's 1954 Attributes

We shall below systematically compare a series of other Midtown II Panel characteristics with those of two appropriate kindred populations. But before venturing into such group comparisons, the reader may properly ask for a "get acquainted" close-up of our 695 Panel subjects, as they would have appeared to us in their fleshed-out social particularities had they assembled on the capacious Radio City Music Hall stage in 1954, that is, before their geographic dispersal.

In table 2.3, the Panel has registered its distributions on five sets of characteristics. The gender ratio at first glance seems unusually unbalanced, in a male to female sex ratio of 1.00 : 0.73. However this is not a sampling idiosyncrasy: the U.S. Census Bureau reported a 1.00 : 0.79 sex ratio for the Midtown area in 1950, and 1.00 : 0.72 sex ratio in 1970.[20]

In age composition, the Panel is spread across a broad midstream span, with a smallish normal-curve "bulge" in the central age cohorts (*B* and *C*).

A similar kind of statement can be made for the Panel's socioeconomic antecedents. Here the distribution also approximates a normal curve (around the modal—highest frequency —lower-middle stratum), except for the small bulge of the top-most stratum. The latter reflects the post-World War I pull of Manhattan's affluent elements into Midtown's most preferred residences.

However, the normal curve statistical figure-of-speech does not do justice to a parental socioeconomic range that in asset terms actually stretched from the near-poorest families to the near-richest in the land. It may be even more illuminating to focus directly on the Panel's subjects in their 1954 specific occupational niches.

The men panned across the spectrum of day laborers, factory operators, skilled artisans, shopkeepers, office and sales personnel, junior and senior executives, graphic and performing artists, writers, lawyers, physicians, and laboratory scientists. The part- or full-time working women (including 53 percent of the wives) were similarly a great miscellany: charwomen, servants, seamstresses, factory operators, beauticians, secretaries, office managers, social workers, nurses, teachers, magazine editors, and social scientists.

Occupying one hierarchical extreme were eight subjects listed either in the City's elite *Social Register* ("Blue Book") or *Who's Who in America*. At the other extreme were fifty-four families on the pre-1954 rolls of the City's Welfare Department, or on the records of the municipal courts or social service agencies.[21]

The Panel's mixture in attained level of schooling reflected American history in the strong upward push of its education escalator. Earlier in this century, the modal schooling level among American whites consisted of people who had not gone beyond the elementary grades; by 1954 the Panel's modal position had been preempted by the high schoolers, with nearly an equal number at the levels of college and above.

The Panel's scatter across the whole Generation-in-U.S. spectrum highlights the successive layers of generations sprung from the immigrants who made New York City, and in particular Manhattan, their principal port of entry and first area of settlement.

Not shown, but cutting across the entire Generation-in-U.S. succession were those identified with origins in the three major religious communities, in descending order of numerical prominence—Catholic (45.0 percent, Protestant (33.6 percent), Jewish (15.8 percent), and Other (5.6 percent).

Also traversing generations *A*, *B*, and *C* were groups of differing national provenance, drawn from across the entire European continent, stretching in an arc from the banks of the River Shannon to the Russias, with the largest number from Ireland and "Mittel Europa."

Pre-1954 History Encountered by the Midtown Panel

In retrospect, at the threshold of the first mass immigration wave of the 1850s, the white population had been culturally Anglo-Saxon Protestants in the main. A century later our Midtown Panel exhibited the enormous sociocultural proliferations that had burgeoned since the post-Civil War industrialization and the immigration waves of the late-1890s, when our first prospective panelists were born.

All in all, this country has elaborated and incorporated into its original Anglican heritage many diverse strands, to a degree probably unmatched anywhere else, weaving a multicolored, patchwork fabric, of a design first labelled "cultural pluralism" by the American philosopher Horace Kallen.[22] Perhaps nowhere in its continental expanse had this conglomerate been more fully developed than in its largest city. Midtown, as an inner-city enclave of that metropolis, contributed its patchwork complexity to the Study's sample of 1954, and ripened by time, to its reinterviewed Panel of 1974.

The people we have just reviewed "close up" can also be likened, in another kind of metaphor, to the equivalent of an evolutionary "mini-Grand Canyon," one exposing a geological-like cross-section of layer upon layer of national experience accumulated since the turn of the century at one of the continent's gateways to the Western world.[23]

To document some of the "historical experiences" just referred to, we asked our panelists to flash back to their 1941–1945 years. Their answers revealed that 144 of the men (49 percent) and two women were drawn from their well-trodden civilian pathways into the military ranks here or in their country of origin; 90 of these men (62 percent) were in areas of combat fire, with 28 (19 percent) suffering hospitalized injuries[24] and 11 (8 percent) incarcerated, for up to four years, in Japanese or German P.O.W. camps. Several received "total disability" medical discharges. An illustration is the man who descended into chronic incapacitating alcoholism, dating from the decimation of his infantry unit during the bitter wintery Battle of the Bulge. His condition was apparent to us in both 1954 and 1974 (when a daughter helped us to conduct the reinterview).

Viewed from the women's side, 38 percent of them had moved into war-related work, 56 percent had a husband, father, son or brother in military service, 9 percent of those kinsmen were killed, and 10 percent injured. As our most extreme case, one Panel member was a Gold Star mother four times over!

On the other side of that earth-engulfing war was a man who had been brought up in the Hitler Jugend, decorated for combat service, and, when asked in 1974 (as were all Panel subjects) "What was the hardest blow of your life?," unhesitatingly replied "The surrender of Germany!" Echoes, almost three decades after V-E Day, of "Deutschland Über Alles!"

Related to this product of Hitler, in a geopolitical sense, were four men who for years had endured the incessant houndings of the Nazi concentration camps, surviving and coping with the crushing weight of wife, children and other kin left behind in ash heaps, and a tattooed left forearm as mute witness.[25]

All of our panelists in 1954 were only a decade away from what historian William L. Shirer has called "the nightmare years" of World War II, and only two decades away from the depths of the Great Depression, which left about one-fifth of those who were adolescents or older at the time with indelible memories of want.

The Panel Lined Up with Two Reference Populations

Having scrutinized our panelists, as if they had gathered before us in 1954, with their personal ordeals trailing not far behind, the reader will have perceived the myriad range of their pluralistic varieties. The large task still before us in this chapter is to answer this question: Can we demonstrate that their diversities were representative of those of the total of the Midtown I sample, at least of those who were to remain alive by 1974? For this purpose we shall designate the latter as the "Total Sample Survivors," (TSS) and compare them as a "reference population" entity vis-à-vis the Midtown II Panel as a living subsample entity. To conduct the demonstration for the reader we must move to establish the number of Midtown I subjects remaining alive in the TSS aggregate, by first subtracting the 266 verified deceased from the original sample of 1660 Midtowners, leaving a remainder of 1394. Ideally we would also subtract the 100 subjects estimated in table 2.2 as the Unlocated Deceased, that is, were we able to identify them individually for removal to the verified Deceased category. Since it is impossible to pin down their separate identities, we are forced in tables 2.4 and 2.5 to work with a TSS number of 1394, as a close approximation of the "true" estimated number of 1294 sample survivors.[26]

In table 2.4, which follows, the first column replicates the Reinterviewed Panel's figures that appeared in table 2.3, for juxtaposition and "eyeball" comparison with the 1954 distributions (in the two adjoining columns) of the identical attributes among the related Located Alive and TSS aggregates.

To first run down columns 1 and 2 together, it is immediately apparent that in no instance does a pair of adjoining percentages differ by a margin greater than 1.1 percent. As we have observed in the paired geographic percentages of table 2.2, the Panel and Located Alive subsamples, for statistical purposes, are in effect identical twins.

This leaves us with the question of whether in its attributes the Panel sufficiently resembles the TSS to serve as a representative surrogate of the latter? Before deciding, however, we must take into account this caveat: realistically, we cannot expect anything approximating perfect concordance between columns 1 and 3.

First, both groups are spin-offs of the 1954 sample and as such are subject to the predictable, random chance fluctuations that are inevitable in the nature of sampling, fluctuations that are technically referred to as "standard sampling error." It would be going too far afield, here, to explain the mathematics of such fluctuations, except to say (1)

TABLE 2.4
Major Demographic Attributes of the Midtown II Panel
in 1954 and Two Kindred Reference Populations

Attribute:	Reinterviewed Panel (N = 695)	Located Alive (N = 858)	TSS (N = 1,394)
I. Gender			
A. Male	42.3%	41.9%	38.7%
B. Female	57.7%	58.1%	61.3%
II. Decade of Birth			
A. 1895–1894	19.3%	19.0%	21.3%
B. 1905–1914	28.6%	29.3%	27.7%
C. 1915–1924	28.1%	28.4%	25.5%
D. 1925–1934	24.0%	23.3%	25.5%
III. SES Background[1]			
F. Lower Lower	11.5%	12.8%	13.1%
E. Upper Lower	13.8%	14.3%	15.6%
D. Lower Middle	22.6%	23.1%	23.5%
C. Upper Middle	18.0%	17.2%	17.5%
B. Lower Upper	15.7%	14.9%	14.1%
A. Upper Upper	18.4%	17.7%	16.2%
IV. Generation in U.S.			
A. Foreign-Born (F-B)	28.3%	28.7%	34.5%
B. Children of F-B	37.8%	38.2%	35.6%
C. Grandchildren	17.5%	17.1%	14.6%
D. Great grandchildren	16.4%	16.0%	15.3%
V. Years of Schooling			
A. 0–8	22.6%	23.6%	28.3%
B. 9–12	40.1%	40.6%	41.1%
C. 13–16	23.3%	22.9%	21.0%
D. 17 or more	14.0%	12.9%	9.6%

[1] Based on scoring and summing Father's (a) years of schooling and (b) his mid-life occupation.

that they vary inversely with the size of random samples, (2) that the statistical margin of error (a) for the TSS entity is ±3 percent, plus a small ± error for the unexcluded deceased among them, and (b) for the Reinterviewed Panel it is ±4 percent.[27] In effect, any intra-pair difference less than ±7 percent may be due, with calculable probability, to simultaneous chance fluctuations, and cannot be accepted as statistically reliable.

With this statistical prolegomenon for the nonstatistician, a scanning comparison of columns 1 and 3 in table 2.4 reveals that among the twenty pairs of percentages there reported, the two largest are 6.2 percent and 5.7 percent among the foreign-born and the least educated, respectively. This particular coincidence is attributable to the fact that the two categories are largely the same people, who are also most heavily concentrated among the Unlocateds.

Moreover, part of the 6.2 percent under-representation of the foreign-born in the Panel has been generated by an interesting process unexpectedly uncovered by Operation Trace, namely reverse migration of immigrants who, after years of residence here, permanently return to their country of origin. Such repatriated members of our 1954 sample turned up among our Verified Deceased,[28] our Located Non-reinterviewed, and, in one surprising instance among our Residual Unlocateds, a discovery worth sharing here.

Our Midtown I sample included 24 Puerto Rican-born subjects, few of whom were over the age of 45, yet in 1974 all but three were terminally unlocatable. Skeptical about the magnitude of this loss, we checked with two authoritative sources. The first were social scientists knowledgeable about the generality of this particular ethnic group, who reported its large reverse migration to Puerto Rico, attributable in part to the Island's proximity and low flight fares. The second was a publication of the New York City Board of Education, which documented that in the decade after 1955, a total of 73,000 of its Puerto Rican enrollees had transferred to their parental island. There are no comparable figures available from the city's large parochial school system.

The major motivations for reverse migration have been personally revealed by a Midtown II Panel member who came here from a Scandinavian country in the early 1920s. We interviewed her in 1954 at age 50 and in 1974 at age 70; she had been divorced in the interim. As a pretest for a conceivable Midtown III study, the present senior author arranged for a 1984 reinterview with her (at age 80). After a residence of some sixty years, long a naturalized citizen, apparently fully Americanized, she reported that in a week she was returning to her birthplace for (in paraphrase) two special kinds of support in her last years: the emotional support of "kith and kin," and the higher level of medical and social services available to the elderly in her native land.

"The return of the native son" is one of the abiding themes in Western literature from its biblical beginnings, and surfaced with some frequency in the immigrant generation of our Midtown I sample. For the country-at-large, the U.S. Immigration and Naturalization Service tells us that "a third of all U.S. immigrants eventually returned to their na-

TABLE 2.5

Distributions of Three Sets of Major Health Characteristics of
the Midtown II Panel and Two Kindred Reference Populations in 1954

Attribute:	Reinterviewed Panel (N = 695)	Located Alive (N = 858)	TSS (N = 1,394)
I. Self-Rated General Health			
A. Excellent	41.6%	39.4%	36.5%
B. Good	42.1%	43.3%	43.7%
C. Fair	13.7%	14.8%	16.6%
D. Poor	2.6%	2.5%	3.2%
II. Overall Mental Health (Symptom Formation)[1]			
A. Well	22.0%	21.1%	19.8%
B. Mild	42.7%	42.4%	40.9%
C. Moderate	21.3%	21.7%	21.5%
D. Marked	9.2%	9.7%	10.5%
E. Serious[2]	4.8%	5.1%	7.3%
III. Pre-1954 Psychiatric Patient History			
A. Now patient	2.7%	2.8%	2.5%
B. Ex-patient	11.4%	10.6%	10.7%
C. Never Patient	85.9%	86.6%	86.8%

[1] These ratings were made by two staff clinical psychiatrists. Their modus operandi is described in chapter 1.
[2] This category combines the psychiatrists' original small classes of "severe" symptom formation and "incapacitated," their frequencies mainly eroded by mortality.

tive lands." Moreover, thousands of American-born citizens annually emigrate to other places.

There are three other key yardsticks by which to compare the Midtown II Panel with its two larger, kindred subsamples. One conveys how their members initially rated their own "general health"; the second reports how two study psychiatrists independently classified panelists' overall mental health status, on the basis of replies to some 83 interview questions about possible current symptoms of emotional distress. The third yardstick registers the frequency, in each column, of exposure, current, former or never, to a psychotherapist.

Perhaps the most serious question addressed in this chapter is whether the Midtown II Panel was disproportionately drawn from the subjects of 1954 who were in the more favorable reaches of the three health indicators of well-being. Table 2.5 enables the reader to answer this question.

The twelve percentage-pairs in the Panel and the Located Alive columns (1 and 2) for all practical purposes are interchangeable. Viewing next the linked percentage-pairs in columns 1 and 3, the differences are in the same directions as those between the paired percentages in columns 1 and 2, and although wider they are not appreciably so.

We have now guided the reader through detailed comparisons (tables 2.2, 2.4, and 2.5) of our Reinterviewed Panel and two larger kindred subsamples, seeking compositional deviations among them on six sets of demographic variables and three sets of health attributes related to the central pillars of the entire Midtown Longitudinal investigation. Most of the differences observed were slight, and even those wider were not large enough to be statistically noteworthy.

Moreover, there were 126 other attributes of various kinds that were covered in 1954 and 1974. Of them 110 were worded exactly the same, whereas sixteen were worded with minor changes. As with the variables in tables 2.2, 2.4, and 2.5 these were also the object of systematic comparison between the Reinterviewed Panel and the TSS population, with these summary results: Relatively few marginal exceptions aside, the differences between the former and the latter on these 126 attributes were not statistically meaningful, and none were statistically significant when corrected for multiple comparisons.

By way of wrap-up of the above step-by-step dissections, we might offer the following closing empirical observation. It will be remembered that the 1954 sample of 1660 age 20–59 interviewees was found to be representative of the total of 110,000 like-age residents of Midtown. We have now reported our estimate that 1294, or 78 percent, of the original sample are twenty-year survivors, located or unlocated. It now seems plausible to make two clarifying assumptions: (1) the sample's estimated 78 percent survival rate can be applied to the total 110,000 figure of 1954, leaving an estimated 1974 total of 85,800 survivors between the ages of 40 and 79; and (2) on the strength of the detailed tabulations presented above, our 695 dispersed reinterviewees at stage-center of this monograph may be a roughly representative surrogate subsample of the total 85,800 estimated survivors of the original 110,000 Midtowners.

On this basis, it may be inferred that despite the considerable erosions of time among their age-peers of 1954, our panelists conceivably have a generalizable significance for a larger, although geographically unusual, population than we might have originally expected from our difficult but indispensable Operation Trace.

Recapitulation

"Stage Manager" in the play *Our Town* identified Grover's Corners and his cast of twenty-three townspeople in a seven-minute soliloquy. The present chapter was necessary to perform those and related functions for our Midtown II macro-cast of 695 reinterviewed subjects. For a scientific, rather than theatrical, narrative, we have had to go to considerable lengths to disclose to the reader how it was possible to cull from the original age 20–59 sample of 1660 concentrated Midtown Manhattan residents a reinterviewed subsample of 695 geographically scattered subjects, all now older by twenty years. As in a popular play revived after many years, with the original cast somewhat shrunken by the vicissitudes of life, our actors were of intrinsic human interest in their own right, toward answering this question: How did they come through the passage of the years? Those years were marked for them by the middle or later stages of the individual life cycle, passing concurrently with the nerve-rattling, roller-coaster social history of the period, together echoing the familiar phrase in the titles of biographies: "The life and the times of..."

However there was the simultaneous extrinsic scientific interest in the question whether this diminished cast could serve as "stand-ins" for all 1294 surviving members, located and unlocated, of the original company.

To answer these skeptical questions persuasively for research specialists and lay generalists, we opened records on the methods and results of our Operation Trace.

Along the way we took the opportunity to enlarge the reader's image and understanding of the anonymous cast, in terms of the great diversities of their attributes, inherited and acquired, and highlights of their remembered pre-1954 life experiences—snippets of autobiography, so to speak, cut out of their personal exposures to the cataclysms of the 1940s and 1930s.

Some final observations on the primary purposes of this chapter may be in order. The Midtown I corpus of publications, often characterized by phrases like "pioneer landmarks," has had continuing impact visible in the research literature,[30] in part because it went to extraordinary lengths to report its methods fully and critically. In fact one professional reviewer of the Midtown I flagship volume wrote: "The authors are at some pains—they seem almost obsessive-compulsive—to examine the weaknesses and biases of their procedures honestly. Indeed, it may well be as a case study in self-conscious research methodology that this book will have its greatest value; the chapters on [research] design are as subtle in their self-questioning as the musing of a Dostoyevsky character" (Friedenberg 1962: 545–47).

In turn, this chapter's extended account of our strategy, tactics and results in confronting the difficult complications of a sequel investigation may have suggestive implications for planning future longitudinal research.

Our most immediate motive was this: the Reinterviewed Panel as a subsample of Midtown I survivors is the foundation on which rests the entire superstructure of findings presented in the chapters that follow. Indispensable to the durability of that edifice is the solidity of its foundation, as judged by tests of its ability to support projections from the Midtown II Panel data to a larger reference population of which it is a representative part, specifically the 1294 survivors, through the year 1974, of the entire Midtown I sample.

This chapter is a brief documenting those tested credentials.

Afternote

Several procedural standards for longitudinal studies are generally recommended: Although biased imbalances often intrude between the original sample and its offspring subsample, previous investigations have been varyingly reticent about fully exposing and assessing them for the reader. Such casual "cover-up" is sometimes veiled by the ruse of reconstructing the subsample with "weights" applied to compensate for the missing subjects, i.e. by arithmetically reconstituting the reinterviewed subsample to make it appear concordant to demographic composition with the parent sample. This cosmetically "corrects" the subsample quantitatively, but evades the question-begging possibility that those most heavily missing from the subsample may be qualitatively different from those who *are* present, on outcome variables crucial to the investigation.

Not only must researchers reveal the extent and nature of major intervening demographic biases, but they are also obligated to report the impact of the latter on their crucial outcome variables. Table 2.5 above especially illustrates this standard, and establishes that the Midtown

Reinterviewed Panel is concordant with its TSS reference population on the key variables of general health, mental health, and psychiatric patient history.

Notes

1. With Anita K. Fischer and Renée Biel.
2. 17 percent of the sample had none.
3. Among investigations conducted with the same people over time from a fixed starting point, a distinction is often made between an aggregate observed for a relatively short term, usually called a "panel," and one followed for a longer period, called a "cohort." For Midtown II's restudied subjects we shall use the former designation, especially as we must refer to the constituent age groups as "birth cohorts."
4. These decisions were especially noteworthy because (1) they were made in a period when longitudinal research was among the lowest priorities of federal funding agencies, and (2) advisory committee members were often themselves partial to short-term study grants. Counteracting these weighty extrinsic considerations was the track record of the Midtown I study as a pioneer of the post-World War II decades.
5. Excluded in some longitudinal investigations have been members of the original sample who had moved beyond the study area's boundaries. Such exclusion, by act of the researchers, can compromise the representative integrity of their remaining subsample.
6. Of course, involved is the standard procedure for one-point-of-time probability sampling, but here extended to, and adapted for, followup of an earlier sample, yielding what is sometimes referred to as a "spinoff" sub-sample. The adaptation was recommended by our eminent advisors on survey sampling, Professor Emeritus W. Edwards Deming of New York University, and Dean Richard Remington of the University of Michigan School of Public Health.
7. Checking out-of-state and out-of-country certificate archives was out of the question on grounds of forbidding cost.
8. Checking the huge, year-by-year files of the decentralized New York City Marriage License Bureau for our missing women turned into a sand-sifting hunt for a husband's surname that, after an unproductive trial-run, was dropped.
9. Single Room Occupancy facility for the indigent.
10. According to the U.S. Census Bureau, 12 percent of the Midtown households in 1950 had lived at a different address the year before. As an independent source of information, our own sample of 1954 (95 percent of them renters at the time) told us that between the age of 18 and the year of interview their stay at each previous address, by our calculation, had averaged 3.5 years overall. Both figures are indicators suggesting something of the momentum of residential turnover in the area that followed after 1954.
11. We feel it may not be inappropriate to share the following empathetic professional observation with the reader: "Longitudinal...studies require a type of patience and care unparalleled in other types of behavioral sciences research. The repeated measurement of a sample of persons for ten to thirty years requires a level of devotion and involvement that is very rare in the annals of research." (Benjamin S. Bloom, *Stability and Change in Human Characteristics*, p.ix. New York: J. Wiley & Son, 1964.)
12. P.D. Scott, "Book Review of Robins, Lee N. 1966. *Deviant Children Grown Up.*

London: E. & S. Livingstone Ltd." In *British Journal of Psychiatry* 113 (August 1967): 929–30.

13. One example is the longitudinal, large-scale national sample survey conducted in Canada, focused on "Quality of Life" indicators. After two years, 66 percent of the subjects were reinterviewed, and 34 percent were lost to followup, including 7 percent who "could not be located," a residual unlocated rate averaging 3.5 percent per annum. Analysis of these unlocatable people, along the lines here applied to their Midtown I counterparts, has not been reported. (See Atkinson 1982: 117.) Another example is an eight-year followup investigation in New Haven, Connecticut that reported a "not located" frequency of 9 percent, or 1.14 percent per annum. (See Regier et al. 1984: 935, table 1.) An earlier example is the 11 percent annual unlocatable rate yielded in the two-year followup of a community sample of San Franciscans age sixty and over. (See Lowenthal et al. 1967: 163.) Unlike Midtown II, the Canadian, New Haven, and San Francisco projects all had the advantages of being preplanned.

14. A Midtown disability case illustration was an unmarried woman who, in 1954, had been patently disturbed but uncommunicative: in 1974 she did not respond to our numerous house calls, and was described by a neighbor in terms suggesting a condition of paranoia: "She comes out only at night, never answers the door, and speaks to no one, not even to a sister, who brings and leaves food at her door step." The most distant case of inaccessibility is the man we traced to the People's Republic of China.

15. Veroff et al. 1981: 29.

16. Sample surveys have consistently yielded rather disparate numbers of the sexes, with the following explanation offered: "The apparent underrepresentation of male subjects is in part due to [the fact] that men are more difficult to locate for interviews." (Regier et al. 1984: 938).

17. This has been a shrinking tendency in recent decades.

18. For consistency with our corpus of Study publications we shall continue to use "the Midtown Panel," with the specification that the phrase refers to its members' 1954 provenance, not necessarily to their 1974 place of residence.

19. The Panel's credentials as a representative subsample that is generalizable to a larger relevant population will be critically examined in all the remaining tables of this chapter.

20. Partially reflected is the fact that work places in the Manhattan Central Business District, which is due south of the Midtown study area, have long been principally "manned" by women settled within easy reach of public transportation.

21. Genealogically not a few Midtowners were from parents or grandparents who had come uptown from the warrens of Manhattan's Lower East Side. Although not a member of our 1954 sample, the renowned popular composer Irving Berlin had himself made the move from the sidewalks of the Lower East Side to the broadwalks of the Upper East Side, a geographic distance of only four miles, but an enormous social class distance denoted by the phrase "rags to riches."

22. Kallen 1924.

23. As a footnote observation: most long-term longitudinal studies in the public health field have chosen to work with panels that were rather homogeneous in age (usually young) or in gender (usually male) or in nativity (usually U.S.-born) or in social class (usually upper or middle). An example of an investigation that was of solid homogeneity in all four of these respects is to be found in the exemplary 30-year followup of 95 purposively (nonrandomly) selected "best and brightest" male Ivy League undergraduates, reported in Vaillant (1977).

24. For the 16.5 million Americans in uniform, including those not exposed to enemy fire, the comparable injury rate was 7 percent.
25. See Levi 1957.
26. In using the "TSS" designation, the quotation marks are intended to remind the reader that approximately 93 percent, rather than 100 percent, of the group are estimated to be alive. This is a deviation probably too small to have more than a minor effect on the TSS distributions in the tables below.
27. This means that one can say with 95 percent accuracy that the results are within plus or minus four percentage points of what they would have been had the entire parent population been similarly surveyed.
28. In one case, verification was made by the burgermeister of the village to which we had traced our subject.
29. For example, a national sample in 1971 was asked: "If you were free to do so, would you like to go and settle down in another country?" Twelve percent replied "Yes."
30. The American Institute of Scientific Information has designated *Mental Health in the Metropolis*, the Midtown I flagship monograph, as a "Citation Classic," on the criterion that it has been quoted in some 1700 surveyed professional books and journal articles. At this writing (1988) the most recent of these pieces appeared in Dumont (1987: 12).

References

Atkinson, Thomas H. "The Stability and Validity of Quality of Life Measures." *Social Indicators Research* 10 (October 1982): 117.

Dumont, Matthew P. "A Diagnostic Parable." *Readings*, American Orthopsychiatric Association, 2 (December 1987): 12.

Kallen, Horace. 1924. *Culture and Democracy in the United States*. New York: Boni and Liveright.

Friedenberg, Edgar Z. Review of *Mental Health in the Metropolis. Commentary*, December 1962, pp. 545–47.

Levi, Primo. 1957. *Survival in Auschwitz*. London: Collier Macmillan Publishers.

Lowenthal, Marjorie F., Paul L. Berkman, and Associates. 1967. *Aging and Mental Disorder in San Francisco: A social psychiatric study*. San Francisco: Jossey-Bass.

Regier, Darrel A., Jerome K. Myers, Morton Kramer, Lee N. Robins, Dan G. Blazer, Richard L. Hough, William W. Eaton, and Ben Z. Locke. "The NIMH Epidemiologic Catchment Area Program." *Archives of General Psychiatry* 41 (October 1984): 933–41.

Vaillant, George E. 1977. *Adaptation to Life: How the Best and the Brightest Came of Age*. Boston, MA: Little Brown & Co.

Veroff, Joseph, Elizabeth Douvan, and Richard A. Kulka. 1981. *The Inner American: A Self-portrayal from 1957 to 1976*. New York: Basic Books.

3

Demographic Aspects of Mental Health

Age Differences, Twenty Years of Aging, Generation-Separated Cohorts of Like Age, and Mental Health Continuity

Among all of the ways in which people may differ from each other, some have been identified by the behavioral sciences as "demographic variables." Such variables have been defined as "culturally significant properties or conditions, differentially manifested by *all* individuals, that provide a basis for classifying a population into a limited series of social segments or groups."[1]

From the start of the Midtown I planning phase, the age of the research subjects engaged the Study team's attention, initially revolving around two questions: What ages should we formally exclude? How should we conceptualize the significance of age for the Study?

We stated our answer to the first question as follows: "In one direction we decided to confine the survey to Midtowners beyond the formative, relatively protected ("teen") years of adolescence, and at least initially launched in the swim of mature life...At the other extreme we decided to exclude adults in the declining years of life, a period when aging and its organic concomitants can complicate the mental health picture and obscure its sociocultural traces. By these boundary definitions the population universe to be sampled was narrowed to people in the prime-of-life range spanning the ages of twenty through fifty-nine."[2] We chose the boundary lines of the U.S. Census Bureau publications that provided national reference norms.

This age range allowed us to compare the average levels of mental health of the Midtowners in four age groups. We assumed that such comparisons would inform us about the health consequences of aging, in a relatively young adult general population. But in a recent review of the period Morton Hunt recalls that "in the early-1950s...the study of aging scarcely existed...Virtually the only attention paid to the subject was the study of diseases in the institutionalized elderly, and the prevailing view of aging was that it was a time of slow and inevitable deterioration, decay, disease and folly."[3]

In Midtown I we had viewed four ten-year age groups within a one-year period. With Midtown II each of these groups taken singly can be studied twenty years older. This allows us to follow a "life-span" approach.[4] We wish to take a modest first empirical step toward formulating both a static and dynamic view of adult age, using an identical yardstick of mental health outcomes in both instances. Our overriding question is: To what extent had each age group changed, and in what ways had each group continued more or less unchanged?

From the Midtown I survey a key summary was that "a substantial process of slippage in mental health seems to mark the path of individual progression through the 20 to 59 age range."[5] With aging seemingly unfavorably implicated, this was our plausible hypothesis: Twenty years of additional aging would be accompanied in our Midtown II panel by further deterioration in mental health. With this in mind we asked the Midtowners for their impression of the trend in the preceding two decades. This was our exact wording: "In your opinion, during the past 20 years have people become more healthy emotionally, less healthy, or hasn't there been much change?" Among those who responded, 11 percent said "Healthier," 76 percent said "Less Healthy," and 13 percent saw "Not Much Change."

This majority opinion was perhaps influenced for some by the poet W.H. Auden's comment that "this is the Age of Anxiety," and for others by a somewhat differently worded professional judgment by several prominent psychiatrists to the effect that "we are in an era of melancholy." Our own hypothesis was consistent with these observations. We planned to use the Midtowners' life histories collected in Midtown I to predict and explain the extent of their worsened mental health, while data from the restudy could be used to specify which aspects of their life history since 1954 further predicted this deterioration.

We empirically test that hypothesis by comparing the Midtowners' mental health in 1974 with their mental health twenty years earlier. The expected worsening is not found. On the contrary, a slight overall improvement appears, with a somewhat higher Well rate of 25 percent, up from 22 percent, and a reduced Impairment rate of 12 percent, down from 14 percent.[6]

Note that the great similarity between the two sets of counts does not imply that the mental health status of most individual Midtowners remained the same between Midtown I and II. On the contrary, only about 44 percent were in the same MH grade in 1974 as in 1954, while 26 percent slipped one or more grades, and 31 percent improved one or more grades.[7]

We next study the data portraying the mental health levels of Midtown I's four decade of birth cohorts after the twenty year interval following 1954. First we see in the counts for 1954 that Impairment rates steadily decline from the oldest cohort, born about 1900, to the youngest cohort, born about 1930, matching the trend of the total sample reported in *Mental Health in the Metropolis*.[8] Moving to the counts for 1974 for the same people, we find a parallel trend, except for an identical small shrinkage in Impairment rates among the three oldest groups that results a lesser tendency towards impairment with increasing age than in 1954.

Did older age, then, predict that the Midtowners' MH would be less favorable, both in earlier and later adulthood? This would seem to be the case if the panel's age is simply considered to be the number of years they had been alive, and nothing more. An alternative view of age is to ask if, when the Midtowners in later adulthood had been the same age as those in earlier adulthood, their MH had been at the same average level as those in earlier adulthood.

To answer this question, we extract and compare only the rates for the 40–49 and 50–59 Midtowners from the preceding data. In other words, cohort A at age 50–59 in 1954 is compared with cohort C at like-age in 1974; and cohort B at 40–49 in 1954 is paired with like-age cohort D in 1974. For narrative convenience let us designate cohorts A and B (both of 1954) as the "Earlier" generation and cohorts C and D (both of 1974) as the "Later" generation, the generations having been born twenty years apart. The Later generation is the historical successor of the Earlier generation; when the Later generation was being born the Earlier generation was moving out of adolescence.[9]

We find that compared to the impairment rates of the Earlier cohorts, those of the Later cohorts *at like age* are one half lower, with the differences at a high level of statistical confidence.[10] This finding was totally unanticipated at the time the Midtown II study was planned.

We note that this finding puts the two older (40–59) cohorts of 1954 in a new light by implying that their high MH54 impairment rates primarily reflect not their life-cycle age but their membership in the Earlier generation. This relatively unfavorable legacy accompanies them when they have moved into the geriatric 60–79 age bracket in 1974.

In this manner we view age as a dynamic aspect of how adults living at the same time and broadly ranging in age are representative of different historical eras, rather than representative of the same historical era but simply for different periods of time (the static view of age). The Midtowners who were 60–79 in 1974 were not representatives of the same historical era as the Midtowners who were 40–59 in 1974, but simply for twenty years longer; they were most importantly of a different, earlier historical era who happened to be alive twenty years longer than their successors.[12]

Genders, Marital Status, and Mental Health Over Time

These intriguing findings led us to search for other demographic variables which might predict MH, beginning with the genders and their various pathways into and out of marriage.[13]

In one respect, dealing with two categories, like males and females, is statistically easier then dealing with twice the number of age cohorts, especially as we must continue to take the latter into account. In other respects our tasks here are far more complicated. To begin with, the biological differences between men and women contribute to their taking partially diverging social roles. Furthermore, the third quarter of the twentieth century, the period of the Midtown Studies, was marked by accelerating development of the genders' role-careers.[14]

Finally, on the pivotal subject of health among women, a recent definitive work has concluded that "the relative influence of nature, nurture and social structure on [their] health outcomes is an area only recently opened up to research by social as well as biological scientists, and a large part of the evidence is not in or is in dispute."[15]

With specific respect to MH differences between the genders, the evidence is somewhat equivocal. To be sure, most studies on this variable have reported more unfavorable findings for females. For example, about four years before Midtown II a nationwide sample investigation was conducted by the federal National Health Examination Survey. Using an interview battery of twelve symptoms of emotional disturbance, it was found that "women had significantly higher rates for every symptom."[16]

Critics of this frequently documented gender difference have argued that it may be an artifact of two opposite gender-linked response tendencies: (1) the culturally rooted "macho" tendency of men to delay admitting psychic distress, and (2) the open sensitivity of females to the biological ups and downs of their menstrual and reproductive cycles. Stated differently, the female is more acutely tuned to signals from her inside body than the male (Martin 1987). The relative salience of these tendencies has remained difficult for research to resolve. We shall simply report our evidence on gender differences among the Midtowners, with no further reference to considerations beyond the scope of our studies.

In Time 1 the impairment frequency of the Midtown women was double that of their male neighbors, anticipating the consensual findings of other community population research that was to follow. Twenty years later the rate for Midtown men remained unchanged, whereas surprisingly the rate for Midtown women had fallen by more than one third.[11] This warrants several comments: (1) the small reduction in impairment cases reported in the preceding chapter was almost completely accounted for by the women; and (2) the panel women as a group are somewhat older than the men: In the two oldest age cohorts (A and B) are 34 percent of the women but only 26 percent of the Men.

In the "Sex and Marital Status" chapter of the *Mental Health in the Metropolis* monograph, the Study team was lured by the observed age trends to bypass this analysis and to proceed directly to the summary statement that "in no age group is there a statistically significant sex difference."[17] In fact the Midtown women were more than twice as likely as the men to have Impaired MH in 1954, a larger ratio than expected by chance alone.

There are enough Midtown women (N=401) to study their impairment percentages of 1954 and 1974 in each of the four birth cohorts. We find that the twenty-year reduction in mental health impairment, found to be confined to the panel women, is diluted when they are combined with the panel men in their joint cohorts, so that the overall inter-cohort differences are levelled down.[18] We can now make intergender comparisons of generation-separated pairs of like-age (40–49, 50–59) cohorts. Those who expect that the Midtown women of the Later generation will have a higher rate of MH impairment than their generation's men, relative to the preceding generation at like-age, will find no support. When we examine cohort A's data, at age 50 to 59 in 1954, we find that the Impaired frequency is 15 percent for its men, and an appreciably higher 26 percent for its women. However we then encounter cohort C, at like-age (50 to 59 years) in 1974, where the Impaired rates for its two gender groups have both dropped from cohort A's levels, but with a significantly greater decrease among the women, down to about the same level as the men.[19]

Turning now to each gender in cohorts *B* and *D*, at age 40 to 49 years, a comparison of the genders reveals the same pattern of changes in impairment from the Earlier to the Later generations; the male-female disparity (9 percent and 21 percent) in earlier cohort *B* becomes the male-female similarity (9 percent and 8 percent) in the like-age, but later, cohort *D*. It seems, therefore, that shifts in individual MH status balance out at net in the same way for the panel's sexes. Nevertheless, time as the procession of generations is more favorable to the Midtown women's mental health than to that of the Midtown men of the same stage in the life-cycle. These unexpected diversities come as cases of further serendipity.

We recall from our chapter 2 discussion of the pre-1974 Trace operation that among our unlocatables in the 1954 sample were a disproportionate number of unmarried women (mostly 20 to 39 years of age), most of whom probably soon married, changed surnames and addresses, and thus were hard to find. Their MH was then appreciably more favorable than that of their single male age-peers (Srole 1962: 178). Hence, had we been able to locate them as successfully as we had the men, these women would probably have had a larger representation in our panel cohorts *C* and *D* (ages 40 to 59 years in 1974), where their presence would likely have produced an even greater intergender MH contrast.

These unexpected gender-linked differences call for a plausible explanation.[20] We shall soon present our statistical efforts to develop one. But first we must follow the genders, so far as possible, into their marital careers, widely reputed to be intimately linked with their mental health status.

Stability and Change in Levels of Marital Status from 1954 to 1974

We know that our panel aged twenty years by 1974: Let us note some changes that occurred in their domestic life circumstances, starting with marital status.

From 1954 to 1974 the Midtowners' marital status can be described as follows:

- Of the 695 Midtowners, 459 (66 percent) were married in 1954. By 1974 348 were still married (76 percent), 85 were widowed (18 percent), 14 were divorced (3 percent), and 12 were separated (3 percent).
- Of the Midtown women, 257 (64 percent) were Married, 60 (15 percent) were Ex-Married (Widowed, Divorced, or Separated), and 84 (21 percent) were Never Married, whereas of the Midtown men, 203 (69 percent) were

Married, 18 (6 percent) were Ex-Married, and 73 (25 percent) were Never Married.

- In 1954 159 Midtowners (23 percent) had never married.

Thus we see that about two thirds of these men and women in the 20–59 age range were married in 1954. About two and a half times more Midtown women than men are ex-married, reflecting the considerably shorter life expectancy of husbands even at this pregeriatric stage of life.

- Of the 159 Midtowners who were Never Married in 1954, by 1974 94 have still never married (59 percent), 55 have married and remain married (35 percent), one is widowed (1 percent), six are divorced (4 percent), and three are separated (2 percent).
- Of the 36 Midtowners who were widowed in 1954, 31 remain widowed in 1974 (86 percent), while five have remarried and remain married (14 percent).
- Of the 24 divorced Midtowners in 1954, 11 are still divorced in 1974 (46 percent), nine have remarried and remain married (38 percent), one is separated (4 percent), and three are widowed (12 percent).
- Of the 17 Midtowners who were separated in 1954, four are still separated (24 percent), six have remarried and remain married (35 percent), four are divorced (24 percent), and three are widowed (18 percent).

Overall of the 77 Midtowners who were ex-married in 1954, 57 (74.0 percent) are ex-married in 1974.

In general, of the 695 Midtowners 350 have the same level of marital status in 1974 as in 1954 (50 percent), and all but two of these Midtowners are married in both 1954 and 1974. Some change in marital status have occurred among the 345 remaining Midtowners (50 percent), 27 percent and 29 percent respectively, or a change rate of about 1.4 percent annually[21]; three-fourths remain on the same marital level as in 1954.

Gender Differences in Stability and Change in Marital Status

When we again examine these same marital status groups in terms of their marital status twenty years later we see that somewhat more than one fourth of each sex has shifted in marital status. At first glance, this seems to suggest a picture of almost identical relative marital stability in both genders.

However a closer look at where the shifters moved from suggests a troubling inference. We first note that twenty years later 12 percent of the Midtown husbands from 1954 were spouseless, and 34 percent of the wives. Almost three times as many women as men had been displaced from their marriages, principally due to the death of their husbands.

Are there compensating shifts in the other two marital status groups? Concentrating only on the Midtown ex-marrieds of 1954, 71 percent of the men and only 13 percent of the women had remarried by 1974. Thus the process of remarriage was predominantly biased for the ex-married men, and highly biased against the women.

Finally, how did the never-marrieds of 1954 fare by 1974? Of the Midtown women who had Never Married up to 1954, twenty years later 75 percent remain Never Married, 20 percent are Married, and 5 percent are Ex-Married, whereas of the men only 41 percent remain Never Married, 51 percent are Married, and 8 percent are Ex-Married. About twice as many women as men remained Never Married. Powerful differential biases were also operating here.

Adding up each of the gender groups, we find that by 1974, when the Midtowners were in the 40–79 age range, the proportion of spouseless men and women totalled 21 percent and 51 percent respectively.

If we divide the genders by age levels we discover how concentrated are the intergender biases in terms of education and income. First, younger Midtown men (aged 20–39 in 1954, 40–59 in 1974) who were ex-married either in 1954 or in 1974 (or both) had substantially higher educational levels than the younger Midtown women. For example, of the Younger men who were ex-married in 1954, 83 percent were college graduates (and some had additional postgraduate education), whereas only 15 percent of the younger ex-married women were at that educational level. Only among the Younger Midtowners who are ex-Married in 1974 is the mean educational level of the men higher than that of the women.[22]

We next estimate that the mean annual income of the Older ex-married Midtown women went down between 1954 and 1974 from about $11,000 to about $8,500, a loss of about 23 percent. In 1974 the average of $8,500 was somewhat above the NYC poverty line for one person. But let's take a closer look at what lies behind that $8,500 average figure. This reveals that 42 percent of the Older female ex-marrieds had an income of less than $4,600. In fact 14 percent had incomes of less than $2,000. All of these were well below the poverty line. So half of the geriatric women who are spouseless were up against the wall of poverty. Some 27 percent of them were in the relative comfort of having incomes above $13,000.

Marital Status and Mental Health

We have seen that the unmarried Midtown women were socioeconomically disadvantaged, in terms of both education and income. Were they additionally disadvantaged in terms of their mental health status? By way of immediate background, one of the most comprehensive current reviews of the literature relevant to us here cites two extensively quoted authorities (Jessie Bernard and William Grove) to the effect that "recent work has gone so far as to suggest that marriage is positively disadvantageous to women's health...these investigators focussed on mental rather than on physical illness" (Giele 1982: 61).

In the preceding discussion we discerned that twenty years of life-cycle aging had only a slight effect on net mental impairment frequencies. However we then encountered the pronounced effect of successive generations of like-age, and it is this dimension of historical time that we shall hereafter primarily emphasize, beginning with marital status.

As prelude, however, unlike the unchanging characteristic of gender,[23] marital status is a transient demographic variable, as one proceeds from singleness into and out of marriage. We dwell on this obvious point only as a reminder that in comparing a marital category at Time 1 and Time 2 some of the original occupants have certainly been replaced at Time 2 by newcomers.

Second, insufficient numbers of separated, divorced and widowed, especially among our panel men, compel us to merge them into a heterogeneous "ex-married" category.

Our gender- and generation-linked findings are as follows: Among Midtown men of both generations there were too few ex-husbands and bachelors to be treated reliably. However the two generations of husbands had almost the same MH impairment rates (roughly 10 percent).

The Midtown women tell us another story. In the Earlier generation all three marital categories (married, ex-married, and never married) had rates roughly between 20 percent and 30 percent. By the Later generation, however, those rates had all fallen to about the 10 percent level observed among both generations of married men.

Certainly, the above frequencies demonstrate that in the Later generation of the Midtown panel the wives are no worse off than either the contemporaneous unmarried women or the married men of middle (40–59) age. In short, our panel women tell a different story than that of the previously cited authorities who considered that "marriage is positively disadvantageous to women's health."

These observations lead directly to observations concerning the impact of socioeconomic status, of which education and income are leading defining attributes, on mental health status.

Static and Dynamic Impacts of Socioeconomic Status on MH

> Change as it may, socioeconomic status [also known as "social class," and SES] is a lifelong motif in the individual's web of daily experience. One of the dominating designs in the vast tapestry of the nation's culture, it also weaves itself into the dreams, calculations, strivings, triumphs and defeats of many Americans from childhood on. (Srole et al. 1962: 210)

These lines introduce the most completely explored social terrain in the curtain-raising Midtown I monograph of 1962. The exploration was guided by a distinction carrying into the present chapter between (1) Parental Socioeconomic Status during one's childhood years (SESPAR), and (2) Own Socioeconomic Status, later, as an adult in 1954 (SES54).[24] The logic of the distinction follows from the adult subject's mental health situation as the Study's "dependent" (synonym: "outcome") variable. Specifically, SESPAR stands to this outcome as the "independent," childhood *antecedent* to the latter as the adult consequence, a straight before-and-after progression. Own SES, on the other hand, stands to adult mental health as a chronologically *concurrent* social setting, the two interacting in a circular and reciprocal manner.

The senior author of the Midtown I monograph noted that previous studies had all focussed on Own SES alone, or its equivalent, but ventured to treat it as chronologically antecedent to adult mental health. In that volume he presented the Midtown I results for *both* SES measures (229), demonstrating that compared to Parental SES, Own SES inflates the linkage to adult mental health, leading to the decision to confine the rest of the analysis almost exclusively to Parental SES. We follow that precedent here.[25]

The Midtown I data led to the following hypothesis about the lowest reaches of the Parental SES range "wherein those handicapped in personality or social assets from childhood on are trapped as adults at or near the poverty level, there to find themselves enmeshed in a web of burdens that tend to precipitate (or intensify) mental and somatic morbidity; in turn, such precipitations propel the descent deeper into chronic, personality-crushing indigency."

Accordingly, it was the senior author's original anticipation that the Midtown Time 2 follow-up would at least confirm the Time 1 differential disadvantage of Low Parental SES. In doing this analysis we note that with 695 Midtown II panelists, age and gender controls compel us to consolidate the SES range into three categories that are, of course, open to subsample chance fluctuations. We observe that for both genders and both age cohorts the Impaired/Well ratios increase considerably as SES goes from upper to lower. The discriminatory process markedly continues to operate against the Midtowners of Low SES origins.[26]

We also compare the occupants of each stratum in 1954 with themselves two decades later. Starting with the men, across all three SES strata, we discern slight twenty-year improvements (i.e., the minus differences) among the High and Middle strata, and, to our surprise, improvements two or three times larger in the Low stratum of both age cohorts.

For the women a similar surprising pattern emerges, with the Low SES improvements in both age cohorts far larger than those of their male SES peers just mentioned.

To sum up, we began by reporting a twenty-year I/W shrinkage from 65 to 47. We then reported a negligible twenty-year change among the panel men (48 to 38) and a substantial improvement among the women (77 to 54). And as climax, we just reported that most of that improvement is in the lowest third of the Parental SES spectrum. In short, both gender groups contradict our implied Midtown I expectation that time would bear most heavily against the mental health chances of people at the bottom of the social class pyramid.[27]

We are offered an even longer time perspective by next confining ourselves to successive generations of the middle (40–59) aged. In the Earlier generation of women the ratios of all three SES groups are substantially larger than those of males of corresponding SES levels. Moving to the Later generation, we note that the ratios of females of all three SES groups are now approximately the same as those of the males of the like SES stratum.[28] Thus in the perspective of successive generations, women of *all* SES levels in the Later generation have advanced to virtual I/W parity with males in the same generation. To be emphasized, also, is that although substantially outpaced by the Low stratum females, the new age 40–59 generation of middle and high SES women have at least registered a modest I/W advance over mothers who preceded them.

All in all, the dynamic perspective of successive generations of like-age—born before and after the great divide of World War I—strongly highlights the Parental SES differences that surfaced after a twenty-year passage of the decade-of-birth cohorts. With the variable of biological age controlled, these generation differences reflect the diversity of influences embedded in sequential stages of post-1895 history, the year our first Midtown panelists were born.

That the overall linkage of social class and emotional health uncovered in our 1954 Midtown sample, and projected here in 1974, continues to prevail has more recently been documented:

> One of the most consistently documented findings in epidemiological research deals with the inverse relationship between socioeconomic status and mental health. Simply stated, individuals in the lower end of the status spectrum have been found to experience significantly more psychological distress than do individuals higher up on the socioeconomic ladder. (Lin et al. 1986: 249)

In the nationwide Epidemiological Catchment Area (ECA) survey of specific DSM-III disorders (Regier et al. 1984), Holzer et al. (1986) report as well that disadvantaged SES is a strong risk factor for alcohol abuse or dependence and antisocial personality disorder, and a weak but statistically significant risk factor for Major Depressive Disorder. Bruce et al. (1993) present data from the one-year follow-up component of ECA showing that disadvantaged SES is a risk factor for the incidence of specific types of psychiatric disorders. A very recent specific test of "the social causation-social selection issue" in "socioeconomic status and psychiatric disorders" is presented in Dohrenwend et al. (1992). Kessler et al. (1995) show that psychiatric disorders have a large and negative effect on educational attainment, a major component of SES. Williams (1993) summarizes the large body of evidence linking SES to health status, including psychological distress. Link and Phelan (1995) argue that disadvantaged SES should be considered "a fundamental cause of disease" including psychiatric disorder and psychological distress. McLeod and Shanahan (1993) present longitudinal data associating "poverty" with unfavorable parenting practices and children's psychological distress. Kessler and Magee (1994) focus on persistent violence in the childhood household as a predictor of adult depressive symptom formation. McLeod and Kessler (1990) argue that disadvantaged SES renders adults more vulnerable to "undesirable life events."

This continually expanding body of scholarship attests to the importance of the findings presented in MHIM more than three decades ago.

Notes

1. MHIM 1962, p. 17, here put in the plural.
2. MHIM 1962, p. 33.
3. Hunt 1985: 201–3. That reviewer adds: "In the 1950s longitudinal studies lasting more than a couple of years were not well thought of; they had proven hard to sustain, and longitudinal methodology was still primitive and full of pitfalls. Few social researchers foresaw that over the next twenty-five years long-term research, despite its drawbacks, would come to be seen as the best way to investigate some phenomena and the only way to explore some others" (ibid., p. 202.)
4. The development of this approach to the study of adult lives, beginning with its roots in early childhood, is well documented, e.g., in Lidz (1968) and Offer and Sabshin (1984).
5. Srole 1962 op.cit.: 109.
6. See the Statistical Appendices for supporting tables and figures.
7. See Appendix A in the Statistical Appendices.
8. Remember that the mental health measure for the total sample was the psychiatrists' ratings, whereas for the Restudy panel it is the multiple regression-derived simulation of the psychiatrists' ratings.
9. Simonton (1990: 35) cogently explains the rationale for defining twenty-year age groups as generations.
10. In 1954 the Midtowners of Cohort A, then aged 50–59, had a MH impairment rate of 22 percent, whereas in 1974 the Midtowners of Cohort C, then also aged 50–59, had a MH impairment rate of 10 percent. The difference of –12 percent is statistically significant (p < .01). On the other hand, whereas Cohort B, aged 40–49, had a MH54 impairment rate of 16 percent, Cohort D, aged 40–49, had a MH74 impairment rate of 8 percent. Again the difference, –8 percent, is statistically significant (p < .05).
11. At Time 1 (in 1954) the Midtown men had an impairment rate of 10.5 percent and at Time 2 (in 1974) 9.9 percent. The difference between Time 2 and Time 1 is only –0.6 percent, not statistically significant. In contrast, at Time 1 the Midtown women had an impairment rate of 21.2 percent and at Time 2, 13.2 percent, with a statistically significant reduction of 8 percent.
12. This is the recurring theme of *cohort analysis*, an approach to understanding age-related phenomena as variously influenced by the stage of the life cycle, and the period of history in which persons are born and especially in which they experience their adolescence (Coser 1964: 373). The following is but a small sampling of the research literature in this area: Glenn (1974, 1983); Hannan and Tuma (1979); Klerman, Lavori, Rice et al. (1985); Knoke and Hout (1974); Mason, Mason, Winsborough, and Poole (1973); Mason, Mason, and Winsborough (1974); Nydegger (1981); Riley (1973, 1987); and Rodgers (1982). The sharp controversies surrounding this approach are evident.
13. For a review of the state of sociological knowledge of marriage as of the end of the nineties, see Glick (1990: 139–45).
14. "The 1960s and 1970s were decades of very rapid change in women's lives" (Bianchi and Spain 1986: 6).
15. Giele 1982: 74.
16. Dupuy 1970: 5.
17. Srole et al., 1975: 175. In 1954, the Midtown panel women (N=401) were 128 percent more likely than the Midtown panel men (N=294) to have impaired MH, a statistically significant difference. But in 1974 the same Midtown women were only about 40 percent more likely to have impaired MH than the Midtown men.

Statistical significance in magnitude varies inversely with the size of the samples or subsamples employed. As discussed in chapter 2 of this monograph the Midtown II panel numbered 695 subjects, down from the full Midtown I sample of 1660; in particular the number of men decreased from 690 to 294. When surgically dissecting the latter into eight age-and-sex subgroups in search of fractional impairment rates, chance fluctuations can reduce the remaining numbers below the level of acceptable statistical reliability.

18. This is particularly the case in Cohorts A and D. In 1954, Cohort A of the Midtown women had a MH impairment rate of 26 percent, which dropped to 17 percent in 1974. Similarly, Cohort B women had a MH54 impairment rate of 21 percent and a 1974 rate of 16 percent; Cohort C women a MH54 impairment rate of 16 percent and a 1974 rate of 11 percent; and Cohort D women a MH54 rate of 4 percent and a 1974 rate of 8 percent. None of the differences within the four Cohorts are statistically significant. We are making the point that pooling the genders into one group can hide trends occurring in only one gender.

19. Specifically, in Cohort C the men's impaired rate is 9 percent, which is not significantly different from that of Cohort A. However the women in Cohort C have an impaired rate of 11 percent, which is significantly lower than that of Cohort A.

20. Further statistical data is presented in Appendix B in the Statistical Appendices. The Gender-specific Generation association was first presented by in Srole and Fischer, 1980, op.cit., and caused an immediate sensation in sociopsychiatric epidemiological circles. This article was reprinted in somewhat modified forms several times, attracting substantial amounts of attention at each reappearance.

21. Specifically, 1.36 percent of the men and 1.44 percent of the women annually.

22. Ex-married men had higher educational levels than ex-married women, particularly among the Younger panelists (aged 20–39 in 1954, 40–59 in 1974). Only 16.7 percent of the Younger ex-married men had less than a high school education, and none had simply graduated high school, whereas 53.8 percent of the Younger ex-married women had less than a high school education and 30.8 percent had graduated high school but not completed college. Never Married older women had substantially higher educational levels than their male counterparts. Only among Older panelists did married men have higher educational levels than married women.

    Of the Younger men who are ex-married in 1974, 37.5 percent had college educations, whereas only 17.8 percent of the Younger ex-married women were that highly educated. As was the case with 1954 Marital Status, the Older Never Married women were more highly educated than the men, while the Older Married men were more highly educated than the women.

23. Except for the very small number of people who experience a change in gender.

24. By way of technical specification, SES54 was based on a summation of equally weighted classifications of Midtowner's years of schooling, breadwinner occupational rank, household income bracket, and rental level (as a surrogate indicator of standard of living). SESPAR was based on parallel composite classifications of the Midtowners' fathers' years of schooling and occupational rank; income bracket and rental level were excluded because of the unreliability of the Midtowners' memory for dollar figures after a long spread of time, if indeed they had ever accurately known their father's income level at all. For both SES measures the composite score range was cut into six more or less equally populated groups, that is, equal-interval sextiles, numbered 1–6 from lowest to highest strata, and collapsible when statistically necessary into three classes.

25. The senior author's major scientific interest has always centered primarily on social class strata, and on their discriminatory life outcome chances. We shall

incorporate both SESPAR and SES54 in our life cycle model of MH74 and associated adult outcomes, in later chapters.

26. The specific I/W ratios are as follows: Impaired/Well ratios for men age 20–39 in 1954 decreased from 71 for Low to 47 for Middle to 31 for High Parental SES; for women from 100 to 44 to 20. These ratios declined for men age 40–59 in 1974 from 50 to 39 to 20; and for women from 40 to 36 to 32. For men age 40–59 in 1954 the ratios declined from 80 to 54 to 37; and for women from 314 to 78, and then rose slightly to 92. For men age 60–79 in 1974 the ratios declined slightly from 57 to 54, and then to 30; and for women from 156 to 74 to 37.

27. We shall further explore this surprising trend in our life cycle analyses of adult MH, in later chapters.

28. The specific I/W ratios are as follows: For Earlier men, I/W ratios decline from 71 for Low to 47 for Middle to 31 for Higher; and for women from 100 to 44 to 20. For Later men the ratios decline from 50 to 39 to 20; and for women only slightly from 40 to 36 to 32.

References

Bianchi, Suzanne M. and Daphne Spain. 1986. *American Women in Transition*. New York: Russell Sage Foundation.

Bruce, Martha L., David T. Takeuchi, and Philip J. Leaf. "Poverty and psychiatric status: longitudinal evidence from the New Haven Epidemiological Catchment Area study." *Archives of General Psychiatry* 48 (May 1991): 470–74.

Coser, Rose L., ed. 1964. *The Family, Its Structures and Functions*. New York: St. Martin's Press.

Dohrenwend, Bruce P. "Socioeconomic Status (SES) and psychiatric disorders: Are the issues still compelling?" *Social Psychiatry and Psychiatric Epidemiology* 25 (January 1990): 41–47.

Dohrenwend, Bruce P., Itzhak Levav, Patrick E, Shrout, Sharon Schwartz, Guedalia Naveh, Bruce G. Link, Andrew E. Skodol, and Ann Stueve. "Socioeconomic Status and Psychiatric Disorders: The Social Causation Selection Issue." *Science* 255 (February 1992): 946–51.

Dupuy, Harold J. et al. 1970. "Selected Symptoms of Psychological Distress." National Center for Health Statistics, series 2, no. 37, p. 5.

Giele, Janet Z. 1982. *Women in the Middle Years: Current Knowledge and Directions for Research and Policy*. New York: John Wiley and Sons.

Glenn, Norval D. "Cohort analysts' futile question: statistical attempts to separate age, period and cohort effects (Comment on Mason, Mason, Winsborough, and Poole April 1973)." *American Sociological Review* 41 (October 1974): 900–4.

———. "Age, birth cohorts, and drinking: an illustration of the hazards of infering effects from cohort data." *Journal of Gerontology* 36 (May 1981): 362–69.

Glick, Paul C. "American families: as they are and were." *Social Science Review* 74(3) (April 1990): 139–45.

Hannan, Michael T. and Tuma, Nancy B. "Methods for temporal analysis." *Annual Review of Sociology* 5 (1979): 303–28.

Holzer, Charles E., Brent M. Shea, Jeffrey W. Swanson, Philip J. Leaf, Jerome K. Myers, Linda George, Myrna M. Weissman, and Phillip S. Bednarski. "The increased risk for specific psychiatric disorders among persons of low socioeconomic status." *The American Journal of Social Psychiatry* 6 (Fall 1986): 259–71.

Hunt, Morton. 1985 *Profiles of Social Research*. New York: Russell Sage Foundation.

Kessler, Ronald C., Cindy L. Foster, William B. Saunders, and Paul E. Stang. "Social consequences of psychiatric disorders, I: educational attainment." *American Journal of Psychiatry* 152 (July 1995): 1026–32.

Kessler, Ronald C. and William J. Magee. "Childhood adversities and adult depression: basic patterns of association in a US national survey." *Psychological Medicine* 23 (August 1993): 679–90.
Klerman, Gerald L., Philip W. Lavori, John Rice, Theodore Reich, Jean Endicott, Nancy Andreasen C., Martin B. Keller, and Robert M. Hirschfield. "Birth-cohort trends in rates of major depression among relatives of patients with affective disorder." *Archives of General Psychiatry* 42 (July 1985): 689–93.
Knoke, David and Michael Hout. Reply to Glenn. *American Sociological Review* 41 (October 1974): 905–8.
Lidz, Theodore. 1968. *The Person*. New York: Basic Books.
Lin, Nan, Alfred Dean, and Walter Ensel. 1986. *Social Support, Life Events and Depression*. Orlando, FL: Academic Press.
Link, Bruce G. and Jo C. Phelan. "Social conditions as fundamental causes of disease." *Journal of Health and Social Behavior* (Extra Issue 1995): 80–94.
McLeod, Jane D. and Ronald C. Kessler. "Socioeconomic status differences in vulnerability to undesirable life events." *Journal of Health and Social Behavior* 31 (June 1990): 162–72.
McLeod, Jane D. and Michael J. Shanahan. "Poverty, parenting, and children's mental health." *American Sociological Review* 58 (June 1993): 351–66.
Martin, Emily. *The Woman in the Body: A Cultural Analysis of Reproduction*. Boston: Beacon Press, 1987.
Mason, Karen O., William M. Mason, H. H. Winsborough, and W. Kenneth Poole. "Some methodological issues in cohort analysis of archival data." *American Sociological Review* 38 (April 1973): 242–58.
Mason, Karen O., William M. Mason, and H. H. Winsborough. "Reply to Glenn." *American Sociological Review* 41 (October 1974): 904–5.
Murphy, Jane M., Donald C. Olivier, Richard R. Monson, Arthur M. Sobol, Elizabeth B. Federman, and Alexander H. Leighton. "Depression and anxiety in relation to social status." *Archives of General Psychiatry* 48 (March 1991): 223–28.
Nydegger, Corinne N. "On being caught up in time." *Human Development* 24 (January-February 1981): 1–12.
Offer, Daniel and Melvin Sabshin, eds. 1984. *Normality and the life cycle: a critical integration*. New York: Basic Books.
Regier, Darrel A., Jerome K. Myers, Morton Kramer, Lee N. Robins, Dan G. Blazer, Richard L. Hough, William W. Eaton, and Ben Z.Locke "The NIMH Epidemiologic Catchment Area Program." *Archives of General Psychiatry* 41 (October 1984): 933–41.
Riley, Matilda W. "Aging and cohort succession: interpretations and misinterpretations." *Public Opinion Quarterly* 37 (Spring 1973): 35–49.
———. "On the significance of age in sociology." *American Sociological Review* 52 (February 1987): 1–14.
Rodgers, Willard L. "Estimable functions of age, period, and cohort effects." *American Sociological Review* 47 (December 1982): 774–87.
Srole, Leo, Thomas S. Langner, Stanley T. Michael, Price Kirkpatrick, Marvin K. Opler, and Thomas A. C. Rennie. 1975. *Mental Health in the Metropolis: The Midtown Manhattan Study*. Enlarged and revised edition. Edited by Leo Srole and Anita K. Fischer. New York: New York University Press.
Weissman, Gerald. 1987. *They All Laughed at Christopher Columbus: Tales of Medicine and the Art of Discovery*. New York: Times Books, Random House Inc.
Williams, David R. "Socioeconomic Differentials in Health: A Review and Redirection." *Social Psychology Quarterly* 53 (Spring 1990): 81–99.

4

Biosocial Antecedents of Mental Health

Having set the stage by describing how mental health levels differed among Midtowners in different levels of social and biological age, gender, marital status, and Parental SES, we proceed to the use of correlations and adjusted correlations (path coefficients, which we also call predictions) to test the propositions of MHIM2. We are constrained by considerations of space and expense from presenting the many tables and figures needed to statistically describe a complicated study such as MHIM2. But this presents the opportunity to discursively present the methods and findings in prose rather than numbers. In so doing, we believe that we shall be making comments which reflect what a statistically knowledgeable reader would make of the correlations and path coefficients.[1]

Since the development of the correlations and path coefficients is a challenging and vitally important research activity, we will phase in our presentation by beginning with a simple analysis: We shall look at the associations of Age level, Gender, and Parental SES with Own SES54. After this orientation, we shall examine the associations of socioeconomic status, Parental and Own in 1954, with adult mental health at Time 1 and Time 2. These simple findings are also important, for they will provide the basis for telling if the additional life-span predictors we shall introduce in the following chapter add to our understanding of adult mental health.

Definitions of Sociodemographic Background and Socioeconomic Status (SES)

The Sociodemographic Background characteristics of the Midtowners are their Age level (AGE), Gender, and Parental SES.[2] Their SES characteristics in 1954 and in 1974 are as follows:

a. The Midtowners' own level of SES in 1954 (SES54), which is a composite primarily of their levels of Education, Occupation, and Income in 1954, and also of their level of Rent in 1954.

b. Each primary element of SES54 is also separately considered as a SES attribute, namely Adult level of Education, level of Occupation in 1954, and level of Income in 1954.

c. In chapters following this one, the combination of Parental SES (SESPAR) and SES54 will be considered a measure of SES mobility. This characteristic corresponds to the Midtowners' change in socio-economic status from childhood to adulthood.

We speak of relative *levels* of characteristics, rather than direct measurements of characteristics, because most of the characteristics we are studying were neither precisely defined or accurately measured. Take as an example "Income." Midtowners were asked to choose a *range* of income, on a card handed to them by the interviewer, which best represented their total household income. We did not request their last income tax return, nor did we ask them to specify their household income to the nearest ten dollars (or even thousand dollars). This level of precision (or intrusion) would not be socially appropriate in a household interview focusing on very personal and intimate issues, such as psychological problems, social attitudes, and physical health problems. Nor would it be scientifically appropriate, given that the primary topic of the study was a vaguely defined concept, namely "mental health."

Prediction: The Fundamental Concept of the Findings of Path Analyses

The essential problem addressed by path analysis is as follows:

1. Some characteristic of the Midtowners is associated to various degrees with some of their other characteristics. We call the former the *predicted* characteristic and the latter the *predictors*.

2. But the predictors are associated with each other to various degrees.

3. We would like to know the extent to which one characteristic is predicted by each predictor *as if* those other characteristics were *not at all* associated with each other. The term "prediction" simply means that we have *statistically adjusted* the association between the predicted characteristic and a predictor for the associations among the predictors and their associations with the predicted characteristic.

These questions of which characteristics correlate with each life outcome, and which characteristics predict each life outcome when statistically adjusted, operationalize the vital research questions raised by the propositions of MHIM2.

Path Analysis: Predictions are Adjusted Correlations

In a path analysis we adjust the Pearson correlation between the predicted characteristic and any predictor for the associations among the predictor and the other predictors, and their associations with the predicted characteristic. The adjustment is calculated using multiple regression analysis. These adjusted correlations are often referred to as "path coefficients,"[3] because the correlation between a predictor and the predicted characteristic has been corrected for the paths between the predictor and the other predictors, and their paths to the predicted characteristic.[4] This is best understood with reference to the results of a simple path analysis. Thus we analyze the paths from the Midtowners' Sociodemographic Background characteristics to their level of Own SES.

Predictions of Midtowners' Level of Own SES in 1954 from their Sociodemographic Background

The scientific problem we wish to solve here is the extent to which the Midtowners' levels of each of the Sociodemographic Background characteristics predict their level of SES in 1954, as if the three Sociodemographic Background characteristics were not at all associated with each other. The path analysis of SES54 must account for the following correlations between SES54 and each of the predictor variables:

Age: The low statistically significant[5] correlation indicates that there is a trend for the older Midtowners to have less favorable (lower) levels of SES54.[6]

Sex: There is no trend towards the average SES54 levels of the genders differing from each other.

SESPAR: A strong correlation shows that the more favorable the SES level of the Midtowners' childhood family, the higher is their SES54.

All of these correlations express the degree to which each predictor variable, taken individually, has a significant path to SES54. Age level has a weak path, SESPAR a strong path, and Gender no path at all. The question asked in the path analysis is whether any of these paths change from being significant to being not significant (or vice versa) if the paths connecting the predictors to each other are statistically eliminated from the model, using the controls of multiple regression analysis.

The Midtowners' levels of the three Sociodemographic Background characteristics are associated with each other as follows:

AGE and SEX: There is a low trend towards the Midtown women being, on the average, older than the men.
AGE and SESPAR: There is no trend towards Midtowners of different age levels having different levels of SESPAR.
SEX and SESPAR: There is no trend towards Midtown women having different levels of SESPAR than the men.

The full path analysis answers our question whether any of these paths change from being significant to being not significant (or vice versa) if the paths connecting the predictors to each other are statistically eliminated from the model, using the controls of multiple regression analysis:

The correlation between SESPAR and SES54 is so large, in comparison with all of the other correlations entering into the model, that it is literally impossible for it to be "explained away" (or reduced to statistical insignificance) by controlling the other predictor variables (AGE and SEX). Although AGE is correlated with SES54, when SEX and SESPAR are statistically controlled AGE ceases to be significantly predictive of SES54. The reason is clear: AGE is also significantly correlated with SESPAR. Thus not only do older Midtowners have lower levels of SES in 1954 than the average, they also have lower than average levels of SESPAR.[7] Note that the degree to which SEX predicts SES54 when AGE and SESPAR are statistically controlled remains not significant. Finally we observe that the path coefficient for SESPAR and SES54 is about equal to the correlation before it was adjusted for Age level and Gender. Removing the weak paths among AGE, SEX, and SESPAR, and between AGE and SEX and SES54, has no impact on the strong prediction of SES54 by SESPAR.

We finally come to an "Error" term, which measures the extent to which we have *not* succeeded in predicting SES54 from AGE, SEX, and SESPAR. It reminds us to be appropriately modest[8]: Almost two thirds of the variation in levels of SES54 among Midtowners is "Error" variance (63 percent), so called because it is not associated with any of the predictors in this model. In other words SES54 was only about one-third predictable from the sociodemographic background predictors of age, gender, and level of parental socioeconomic status. We are thus informed that even if all of the Midtowners had come from precisely the same sociodemographic background they still would have had a wide range of levels of SES54.

Why might almost two-thirds of the variation in levels of SES54 be not associated with the predictor variables?

- *Perhaps the model is incorrectly formulated.* For example, the predictors may be influenced by each other in a nonlinear manner, which has not been taken into account in the model. This is called an "interaction" among predictors.[9]

We have observed that the interaction of AGE and SEX does not predict SES54. But perhaps SEX and SESPAR interact to a significant extent; as it happens they do not. Or perhaps the model does not contain some predictor variables it should contain. Note that we choose to only look at the interaction of AGE and SEX for three reasons: (1) There are many possible interactions, so that the models might grow unfathomably complex (2) We know that Age level means something quite different for the Midtown women than for the men, in terms of the progression of generations, as we have seen in the very important case of adult mental health (MH). This interaction therefore has established scientific importance. (3) Furthermore the repeated testing of multiple interactions in the same study magnifies the problem of obtaining "false positive" results from statistical significance tests, that is, of incorrectly concluding that path coefficients are significant when in fact they are not.

- *The predicted variable is imprecisely measured.* As an example of measurement error, income was identified by Midtowners on a card, as described above. This was somewhat vague and imprecise, and drives up Error. We already know, and can observe in our model, that the Midtowners in all different age and gender groups experienced substantial social mobility, thus limiting the extent to which their SES54 can be predicted from their SESPAR. MHIM1 emphasized the "Goldcoast" nature of the Midtown Manhattan study area in 1954.[10] This social process underscores the scientific importance of exploring the predictive value of social mobility with respect to adult functioning twenty years after the baseline study.

We now present analyses which address the predictions of SES54 made by AGE and SESPAR in the Midtown women and men separately.[11] By performing analyses of the data for each gender separately, we learn the extent to which the predictor variables have paths to SES54 only among either the Midtown men or women, but not both.

Sex-Specific Predictions of Midtowners' Own SES in 1954
By Age and SESPAR

We begin by observing the following correlations:

- Among the Midtown women, AGE and SESPAR are not significantly correlated. The older women had slightly lower levels of SES54. The strong association of SESPAR and Own SES54 showed that the higher was their Parental SES, the higher is their Own SES54.
- Among the men, AGE and SESPAR are also not significantly correlated while SESPAR and SES54 are moderately to strongly correlated. Unlike the case with the women, AGE and SES54 are not correlated.

We now compare the predictions of SES54 made by AGE and SEX for the Midtown women with those made for the men:

- Only among the women is there a low trend for the older Midtowners to have less favorable levels of SES54 than the younger Midtowners.
- SESPAR strongly predicts SES54 significantly in both the men and women, and to about the same degree.
- AGE and SESPAR predict about 31 percent of the SES54 in the men and about 41 percent in the women.

Now that we've seen the products of a predictive model of SES54 in the total panel of Midtowners and in each gender group separately, we are ready to approach the prediction of adult mental health in the same manner, and explicitly test the basic propositions of MHIM2.

Predictions of 1954 Mental Health
by Sociodemographic Background

We now test a basic proposition of MHIM2 using the MHIM1 data, simplified as suggested in chapter 1, that Age level, Gender, and Parental SES predict Mental Health in 1954.

In the total sample both the Midtowners' levels of Parental SES and the interaction of AGE and Gender predict their level of Mental Health in 1954. The higher was their SESPAR, the more favorable is their MH54. Although we expect the interaction of AGE and Gender to be significant on the basis of the demographic data presented in chapter 3, we still note as a new finding that it remains significant even when SESPAR is controlled. Only five percent of MH54 is predicted by this model, a slight amount which we remind the reader is still statistically significant (greater than by chance alone).

Among the Midtown women there was a trend for the older subjects to have less favorable levels of MH54 than the younger subjects. But among the men Age did not predict MH54. Among both the men and the women separately, there was a trend for Midtowners with more favorable levels of SESPAR to have more favorable levels of MH54 than Midtowners with less favorable SESPAR. The model predicts six percent of the MH54 in the women, but only one percent in the men, an amount not significantly different than none at all. This substantiates a basic proposition of MHIM2.

Predictions of 1974 Mental Health by Sociodemographic Background and 1954 Adult Functioning

We now test another basic proposition of MHIM with MHIM2 data, that Age level, Gender, Parental SES, and Own SES in 1954 will predict Mental Health in 1974, controlling for Mental Health in 1954. This is our first long-range path analysis of adult mental health twenty years after the baseline study, in 1974.

Methodological Considerations

We have two sets of predictors which have existed in distinctive, but overlapping, segments of the Midtowners' life cycles:

1. The Sociodemographic Background predictors, all of which were established from when the Midtowners were born, which are Age level, Gender, and Parental SES.
2. The 1954 Adult Functioning predictors of 1954 MH and 1954 SES.

Because these two sets of predictors have such clearly different time frames, we solve the model in three different ways, as indicated by the propositions we are testing:

1. We begin by measuring the paths of the predictors furthest in time from the Midtowners' level of MH in 1974 (MH74), the Sociodemographic predictors, controlling for each other; and then measure the paths of the predictors closest in time to MH74, the 1954 Adult Functioning predictors, controlling for each other and for the Sociodemographic predictors. When we control a predictor for its associations with other predictors in the same place in the model, that is with the same temporal reference, we say we are controlling it for *concurrent* predictors. However when we control a predictor for its associations with other predictors which have an *earlier* beginning in the model, we say we are controlling it for *ante-*

cedent predictors. No predictors are antecedent to the Sociodemographics, while the Sociodemographics are antecedent to the 1954 Adult Functioning predictors. Our acronym for this way of solving a path model is "AC."

2. Alternatively we may begin by solving the model first for the predictors which are closest to the predicted characteristic in time, controlling for each other; and then solving the model for the predictors which are more remote from the predicted characteristic, controlling for both each other and for those which are closest to the predicted characteristic in time. When we control a predictor for its associations with other predictors which have a *later* beginning, we are controlling it for *intervening* predictors. No predictors intervene between the 1954 Adult Functioning predictors and MH74, while the 1954 Adult Functioning predictors intervene between the Sociodemographics and MH74. We abbreviate this solution of the model as "IC".

3. Lastly we may solve the model adjusting the path of each predictor to MH74 for its associations with all of the other predictors (and their paths to MH74). We tag this the "AIC" solution, because each predictor is controlled for antecedent, intervening, and concurrent predictors.

Each solution constitutes an armchair experiment of scientific interest. When significant paths are found in one solution, but not another, scientific implications are raised:

1. When a predictor significantly predicts MH74 when only concurrent predictors are controlled, but not when intervening predictors are also controlled, we may infer that the significant prediction is accounted for (or explained) by the predictor's associations with one or more intervening predictors.

2. When a predictor significantly predicts MH74 when only concurrent predictors are controlled, but not when antecedent predictors are additionally controlled, we may infer that the significant prediction is accounted for by paths to it from one or more antecedent predictors. The scientific importance of this result is that the predictor may contribute to explaining the predictions made by the antecedent predictors.

3. When a predictor has a significant path to MH74 when all other predictors are controlled, we can be certain that it in and of itself predicts MH74.

Findings

Let's see how these theoretical considerations apply to the problem at hand, that of predicting MH74 by first the Sociodemographic Background predictors and then by the 1954 Adult Functioning predictors controlling for their paths to the Sociodemographic Background predictors. We'll begin by examining the correlations to see the extent to which each predictor is associated with MH74 before being included in our model.

- The more favorable the Midtowners' level of MH in 1954, the more favorable it is in 1974, a prediction of medium strength.
- There is a trend for Midtowners with more favorable levels of SES54 to have more favorable levels of MH in 1974 (MH74) than Midtowners with less favorable levels of SES54.
- There is also a trend for the older Midtowners to have less favorable levels of MH74 than the younger Midtowners.
- There is no trend for the Genders to significantly differ in their average level of MH74, although there was such a trend for MH54.
- There is a trend for the Midtowners from more favorable SESPAR levels to have more favorable MH74 than the Midtowners from less favorable SESPAR levels.

We continue with the AC path analysis. The younger Midtowners, on the average, have more favorable levels of MH74 than do the older Midtowners. The higher is the Midtowners' SESPAR, the more favorable is their MH74. The Midtowners' gender does not predict their MH74. The more favorable is the Midtowners' MH54, the more favorable is their MH74. There is no trend for Midtowners with different levels of SES to have different levels of MH74 with MH54 and the Sociodemographic Background predictors controlled.

What is the scientific meaning of these findings? We can conclude that the stability of mental health over twenty years of adult life is about medium in strength, after the association has been adjusted for Sociodemographic Background and SES54. Furthermore we conclude that the association of SES54 and MH74 is explained by its associations with MH54. We propose that the Midtowners' level of SES in 1954 contributes to explaining the prediction of their level of MH in 1974 by their level of Parental SES: when we control for SESPAR background, SES54 ceases to predict MH74. Another contributor is of course MH54. However we also find that MH74 is more *not* predicted by the predictors than predicted: only about one fifth of MH74 is predicted by this model (21 percent). We must be appropriately modest, therefore, in claiming to have predicted the Midtowners' levels of MH74, although our model certainly is more successful in predicting MH74 than would be expected by chance alone.

We continue with a path analysis that adjusts each predictor for its associations with intervening and antecedent predictors (IC). This model specifies that the Midtowners' MH54 makes a moderate to strong positive prediction of MH74 whereas their SES54 makes a weak prediction. None of the Sociodemographic predictors have a significant path to MH74. It is a mathematical necessity that the final result of this model is also that it predicts only 21 percent of MH74; the difference between AC and IC (and AIC) is only in the type of controls applied to the predictors, and not in the final percent of predicted variation.

The scientific meaning of these additional findings is that the associations between MH74 and the three sociodemographic predictors are accounted for by the paths from the sociodemographic predictors to the 1954 Adult Functioning predictors. In the case of SESPAR, we find that it stops predicting MH74 when we control for SES54 (and of course MH54). This seems to contradict our finding in the AC model, but actually describes how differently the two models operate. The fact that we observe both of these paths implies that the Midtowners who had more favorable levels of SES54 than SESPAR did not consistently have more favorable levels of MH74, when MH54 is also controlled.

Finally we examine a path analysis in which each predictor is controlled for all of the other predictors (AIC), only to find that the Midtowners' MH54 moderately predicts their MH74, net of the other predictors. The two socioeconomic status variables, SESPAR and SES54, cancel out each other.

It would be scientifically invalid to conclude that socioeconomic status does not predict MH74 from this result. We recall that the Midtowners' Parental SES strongly predicts their SES54. It is not surprising that neither has a significant path to MH74 when the other is controlled, because we are simultaneously discounting the prediction by SESPAR of MH74 for the fact that it predicts SES54 *and* discounting the prediction by SES54 of MH74 for the fact that it is strongly predicted by SESPAR.[12] Therefore we conclude that socioeconomic status is "overcontrolled" by including both of these substantially correlated measures in the model. Only knowing the results of the AC and IC models allows us to avoid this mistake.

A scientifically valid statistical analysis must therefore include all three solutions of the path model.

Sex-Specific Predictions of 1974 Mental Health by Sociodemographic Background and 1954 Adult Functioning

We begin by assessing the correlations among the women between MH74 and these predictors. There is a trend towards older Midtowners having less favorable levels of MH74 than younger Midtowners. There are also trends for Midtowners with increasingly favorable levels of SESPAR and/or SES54 to have increasingly favorable levels of MH74. Finally MH54 has a strong and positive correlation with MH74.

Among the Midtown men, AGE and MH74 are not significantly correlated, unlike the case with the women. There are some other differences between the men and women. Among the men the correlation of SESPAR and MH74 is weak, positive, and significant but that between MH74 and SES54 is almost medium in strength. But among the women both the correlations of SESPAR and SES54 with MH74 are weak. Finally MH54 and MH74 are more strongly correlated among the women, at a moderate level, than among the men, where it is only weak to moderate.

The AC model in the women shows that both AGE and SESPAR have significant and weak paths to MH74. MH54 has a significant and positive path of medium strength to MH74 whereas SES54 does not predict MH74. About one quarter of MH74 is predicted by this model in the women (24 percent).

The IC model in the women makes only one statistically significant prediction: the more favorable the women's level of MH54, the more favorable is their level of MH74, a strong and positive prediction. This also is the sole prediction made by the AIC model in the women.

The AC model in the men works differently than in women: Unlike the case with the women, only SESPAR—and not AGE—has a significant path, positive and weak, to MH74. Again unlike in the women, both MH54 and SES54 have significant paths to MH74 in the Men: MH54 makes a positive and medium strength prediction of MH74, while SES54 makes a positive and weak prediction of MH74. About one-fifth of MH74 in the men is predicted by this model (17 percent).

The IC model in the men also displays a different finding than that in the women: whereas in both Genders the path of MH54 to MH74 is positive, it is strong in the women but only medium in the men. Furthermore in the men SES54 makes a significant positive, weak prediction of MH74, whereas in the women it does not have a significant path to MH74. This finding persists when the antecedent sociodemographic predictors are controlled as well.

We conclude that whereas the men's SES54 predicts their level of MH twenty years later, in 1974, the women's SES54 does not predict their MH74, when (especially) MH54 and SESPAR are taken into account. This gender difference substantiates a basic proposition of

MHIM2. These minimal models predict almost a quarter of the 1974 levels of mental health in the Midtown women (24 percent), 17 percent in the Men, and 21 percent in the total Midtown panel.

Predictions of Generation-Separated Mental Health by Sociodemographic Background

We measured Mental Health at age 40–59 by selecting the MH54 measure for the Earlier Generation and the MH74 measure for the Later Generation. This measure is termed "Generation-Separated Mental Health at Like Age," abbreviated as GMH. We can analyze this new measure, GMH, just as we have analyzed MH54 and MH74 above, with the understanding that the meaning of associations involving "AGE" actually will refer specifically to social age, that is to say Generation.[13]

The predictions of GMH by the Sociodemographic Background predictors of AGE, SEX, and SESPAR are as follows: we first find that AGE is differently associated with GMH in the two Gender groups. We also observe that the higher the Midtowners' SESPAR, the more favorable is their level of GMH. Among the women, AGE and SESPAR both predict GMH. The Later Generation of the women [40–59 in 1974] has a significantly more favorable level of GMH than does the Earlier Generation [40–59 in 1954]. But among the men only SESPAR predicts GMH: the two Generations of the men have about the same average level of GMH. We conclude that while the Gender-specific Generation prediction of GMH discussed in chapter 3 has been again established in these analyses, persisting despite the control for SESPAR, the prediction by Parental SES of GMH is about the same in both Genders. These minimal models explain about 4 percent of GMH in the women, 3 percent in the men, and 5 percent in the total Midtown panel.

Summary and Conclusions

To this point we have been testing some of the basic propositions of MHIM2, using data which reflect some important aspects of the Midtowners' lives, by statistically modeling their adult mental health status using, in the case of 1954, the biosocial predictors of Age Level, Gender, Parental SES; and in the case of 1974 also the Midtowners' SES in 1954 and their 1954 MH. How well have we done in modeling adult mental health with just these background predictors?

Predicting Mental Health With Additional Biopsychosocial Predictors

The amount of variation in the total sample which we can account for this way is as follows: 1954 adult mental health, 5 percent; 1974 adult mental health, 21 percent—largely due to the inclusion of MH54 as a predictor); and generation-specific mental health, 5 percent. Almost all of the variation in mental health is *not* explained. Contrast this finding with that for own level of socioeconomic status in 1954: about a third of the variation is accounted for in the overall panel of Midtowners simply by the Sociodemographic Background predictors, especially SESPAR. We may well wonder how much more we may predict adult mental health by adding the various biopsychosocial predictors implied by the basic propositions of MHIM2 to our predictive model.

Notes

1. Statistically sophisticated readers can find all of the many numerical details of MHIM2 in the Statistical Appendices (see Preface).
2. Other possible biosocial background characteristics such as Generation in the United States and the Religious Orientation of the Family of Origin, will not be considered in this monograph because, as stated in chapter 1, they had already been shown in *Mental Health in the Metropolis* (MHIM1) to not predict the Midtowners' adult level of mental health in 1954 when Parental SES was statistically controlled. Note that the names of variables are capitalized.
3. Another frequently used term is "beta coefficients."
4. No attempt is made here or in the Statistical Appendices to present the mathematical concepts of multiple regression (or path) analysis. Interested readers may find introductions to this topic of varying complexity in such sources as the following: Alwin and Hauser (1975), Cohen and Cohen (1983), Duncan (1969, 1975), Fischer et al. (1979), Heise (1969), Jencks et al. (1972), Kenny (1979), Land (1969), and Li (1975). A good introduction to the various strategies of constructing predictive models of health status or related life outcomes is presented in Greenland (1989).
5. In general we regard correlation coefficients as statistically significant if the probability of their occurring is equal to or less than 5 in 100, the 0.05 level. Path coefficients are also evaluated in that manner, with the additional criterion that the overall amount of variation explained by the predictors in the path analysis is statistically significant (the "sheltering" strategy of Cohen and Cohen 1983). Statistically sophisticated readers may consult the Statistical Appendices for the detailed presentations of all of the path analyses summarized in this monograph. Our measures are sufficiently precise, and collected from a sufficiently large sample (n=695), to make accurate tests of the null hypothesis of no association, to establish the direction of association (positive versus negative), and to establish whether the magnitude of association is low (i.e. about 0.10), medium (i.e., about 0.30), or high (i.e., about 0.70) (Cohen 1969).

6. We make use of synonyms of our terms for the strength of correlations or predictions as needed. We might for example refer to a weak association as showing a slight trend, or a small difference between two groups, that is, the Genders, which is greater than chance alone.

7. Logically it is clear that SESPAR is a predictor of SES54. When the fact that older Midtowners had less favorable levels of SES in their childhood is statistically removed (along with the negligible role of SEX), the prediction by AGE of SES54 is cut in half and is no longer statistically significant.

8. The percentage of explained variation is measured by the squared adjusted multiple correlation of all of the predictors with SES54. The adjustment removes the amount of variation accounted for in the predicted variable simply by the number of predictors in the model.

9. We measure interaction (say, between AGE and SEX) as follows: First we multiply the two predictors to produce a new predictor variable (AGE*SEX). Then we correlate that new predictor (AGE*SEX) with the predicted characteristic (SES54). Finally, using multiple regression analysis, we discount the correlation of the new predictor (AGE*SEX) for its association with each of its two component variables (AGE and SEX) and their paths to the predicted characteristic (SES54).

10. MHIM1 (Srole et al. 1978) describes this in rich detail.

11. The method is often referred to as stratified multiple regression analyses.

12. The statistician's name for this problem is "multicollinearity" (Cohen and Cohen 1983). It occurs when some predictors are much more highly associated with each other than is generally the case.

13. We chose in our path analyses to use the continuous measure of AGE rather than to dichotomize the Midtowners as being either in the Earlier or Later Generation. By so doing we can statistically control whatever variation there is in MH associated with the relative age of the Midtowners within a Generation.

References

Alwin, Duane F. and Robert M. Hauser. "The decomposition of effects in path analysis." *American Sociological Review* 40 (February 1975): 37–47.

Cohen, Jacob. 1969. *Statistical Power Analysis for the Behavioral Sciences.* New York: Academic Press.

Cohen, Jacob and Patricia Cohen. 1983. *Applied Multiple Regression/Correlation Analysis for the Behavioral Sciences,* 2d ed. Hillsdale, NJ: Lawrence Erlbaum Associates.

Duncan, Otis D. 1975. *Introduction to Structural Equation Models.* New York: Academic Press.

———. 1969. "Contingencies in constructing causal models," in *Sociological Methodology 1969,* edited by Edgar F. Borgatta, 74–112. San Francisco: Jossey-Bass Inc.

Fischer, Anita K., Janos Marton, Ernest J. Millman, and Leo Srole. 1979. "Long-range influences on adult mental health: The Midtown Manhattan Longitudinal Study, 1954–1974," in *Research in Community and Mental Health, Vol. 1,* edited by Roberta G. Simmons, 305–33. Greenwich, CT: JAI Press.

Greenland, Sander. "Modeling and variable selection in epidemiologic analysis." *American Journal of Public Health* 79 (March 1989): 340–49.

Heise, David. 1969. "Problems in path analysis and causal inference," in *Sociological Methodology 1969,* edited by Edgar F. Borgatta, 38–73. San Francisco: Jossey-Bass Inc.

Jencks, Christopher, Marshall Smith, Henry Acland, Mary Jo Bane, David Cohen, Herbert Gintis, Barbara Heyns, and Stephan Michelson. 1972. *Inequality: A Reassessment of the Effect of Family and Schooling in America*. New York: Harper and Row, Colophon Edition.

Kenny, David A. 1979. *Correlation and Causality*. New York: Wiley-Interscience, John Wiley & Sons.

Land, Kenneth. 1969. "Principles of path analysis," in *Sociological Methodology 1969*, edited by Edgar F. Borgatta, 3–37. San Francisco: Jossey-Bass Inc.

Li, Ching C. 1975. *Path Analysis—A Primer*. Pacific Grove, CA: Boxwood Press.

Srole, Leo, Thomas S. Langner, Stanley T. Michael, Price Kirkpatrick, Marvin K. Opler, and Thomas A. C. Rennie. 1978. *Mental Health in the Metropolis: The Midtown Manhattan Study*. Revised and enlarged edition. Edited by Leo Srole and Anita K. Fischer. New York: New York University Press.

5

Early Life Experiences and Sociodemographic Background

The objectives of this chapter are as follows:

1. To introduce six new potential predictors of adult mental health status derived from the basic propositions of MHIM2.
2. To describe the way in which the Midtowners' early life experiences are predicted by their Sociodemographic Background characteristics, and when appropriate by their antecedent early life experiences.
3. To compare and contrast the predictions of the Midtowners' early life experiences made by Sociodemographic Background characteristics, and when appropriate by their antecedent early life experiences, in each Gender group.

* * *

To this point we have been testing the basic propositions of MHIM2 by statistically modeling their adult mental health status using, in the case of 1954, only the biosocial predictors of Age level, Gender, Parental Socioeconomic Status (SES); and in the cases of 1974, also the predictors of our Midtowners' level of SES in 1954 and their 1954 level of Mental Health. Our success in explaining adult mental health has been quite limited, but we have established a baseline for more complicated models which we draw from the basic propositions of MHIM2. Have we done so well that to introduce further biographical particulars into our model of adult mental health would be a needless complexity? Or, may adult mental health be viewed straightforwardly as a function of the Midtowners' location in an increasingly irrational social system, as measured by their socioeconomic status, and possibly also biosocial age and sex?

Since 1976 our efforts have been focused on discovering additional true predictors of adult mental health status, that is to say, biopsychosocial[1] characteristics of our Midtowners which preceded their attaining an adult mental health status rather than those which occurred synchronously and therefore are *reciprocal* with adult mental health status. A preliminary attempt to produce a more comprehensive biopsychosocial model of adult mental health status was presented by Fischer et al. (1979). We had reason to be dissatisfied with it: (1) no allowance was made for the Midtowners' own level of Socioeconomic Status in 1954 or its components (occupation, education, and income); (2) a variable mapping a domain of adult experience entirely apart from their mental health status was included as a predictor of 1974 Mental Health level, namely the Midtowners' level of Anomia in 1954 (Srole 1956); (3) the 1954 Adult Functioning indices were combined in two factor indices, with the benefit of simplifying the statistical presentation of path analytic findings but at the cost of obscuring the relative importance of each as a predictor of post-1954 adult mental health status.

Despite these shortcomings, the path analyses presented in Fischer et al. (1979) represented a breakthrough for the Midtown Study, for they presented the measures of early life experience which had been developed by the Midtown Study research team of Leo Srole, Anita Fischer, Janos Marton, and Ernest Joel Millman over a two-year period, based upon a twenty-year meditation on the 1954 study by the senior author of this monograph.[2]

Predicting Mental Health: Bridging the Gap from Sociodemographic Background to 1954 Adult Functioning

The subject of Srole's meditation was not how to increase the amount of variation in 1954 Mental Health accounted for by a path analysis, but rather the scientific question of how can we understand the ways in which people of different levels of Age and Socioeconomic Status in childhood come to have different levels of Mental Health in their adulthood. What are the implications of socioeconomically disadvantaged or advantaged family backgrounds for the pre-adult development of our Midtowners? What were the differences before adulthood in the functioning of Midtowners of different Genders and Generations?

To answer these questions required studying the contexts within which the Midtowners functioned before they became adults. In other words the Midtowners' levels of their Sociodemographic Background characteristics perhaps were predictive of their mental health status as adults because (1) they were first predictive of important aspects of the particular biopsychosocial environments within which they grew up, and (2) they were perhaps also predictive of how well the Midtowners functioned before adulthood in whatever particular biopsychosocial environments they developed. At the same time there may well be aspects of both childhood settings and how favorably the Midtowners functioned before adulthood which are not predicted by their Sociodemographic Background characteristics, and which do predict their adult functioning. All of these issues were derived from the basic propositions of MHIM2.

Additional Predictors

In this chapter we introduce six new measures of the biopsychosocial characteristics of our Midtowners before 1954, including four Contexts of Childhood Functioning, one global measure of Pre-Adult Well-Being, and one composite index of the level of severity of physical health disorders up to 1954 (which includes the adult years preceding the baseline interview). We very much intended to keep our model of Midtowner personal history as simple as possible while at the same time incorporating all of the available information from the 1954 and the 1974 interviews pertinent to testing the basic propositions of MHIM2. To do this we performed many statistical analyses of associations among the individual data items and their predictions of MH. We decided to combine these items into some two dozen measures, and then repeat this process using these measures rather than the individual items. Again we found that we could combine smaller measures into larger ones to simplify the analyses while using all of the available information in a manner consistent with what we knew about individual psychological, biological and social development.

Finally we arrived at six measures which sufficiently differed in their domains to resist further reduction.

Measures of Early Life Experiences

Most of our measures of early life experiences come from the 1954 baseline interview. One measure comes entirely from the 1974 interview, that of Pre-54 Level of Severity of Somatic Disorders. All of these measures are retrospective; that is, our Midtowners were asked to recall aspects of their life before 1954, reaching back to early childhood. An extensive literature on the shortcomings of such measures exists[3] both in the social scientific and epidemiological fields of research. Although we believe that our Midtowners had a good level of rapport with their interviewers and tried their best to objectively reconstruct their past lives, we must acknowledge the tentative nature of this data. We have been and will continue to be modest in presenting our findings, our conclusions being hypotheses for future research. However we note that psychiatric case histories draw to a very substantial extent on the patients' own retrospective report of their present situation and life history, including family history; psychiatric clinicians are of course encouraged to consult past medical records and interview family members and other close associates of their patients. With these caveats, here are our measures of early life experiences, as reported in Fischer et al. (1979):

Body Damage (Context of Childhood Functioning)[4]

We used three items from the 1954 baseline survey to measure Body Damage:
"As far as you know were you born with any physical condition that needed correction?"
"Before the age of 20, did you ever have a heart condition?"
"Did you ever have epilepsy?"
A score of one was received by eighty-six Midtowners, whereas a score of zero was received by the remaining 609 Midtowners.

Parental Intrafamily Functioning
(Context of Childhood Functioning)

Twenty items from the 1954 interview were aggregated to form a global measure of how adequately the Midtowners experienced their parents as having functioned when they were growing up. We looked at two domains of parental functioning within the household, namely their physical health and their role functioning:

1. Midtowners reported whether or not their father or their mother had any of the following ten disorders: arthritis, asthma, bladder trouble, colitis, diabetes, hay fever, high blood pressure, sciatica or neuralgia, stomach ulcer, or a skin condition. These reports were summed to form a measure of Parental Psychosomatic Conditions.
2. The other ten items from 1954 include:
    "When you were growing up (ages 6–18) were either of your parents (parent substitutes) in poor health?"

"Were either of your parents (parent substitutes) the worrying type?"
"Did either of your parents (parent substitutes) have a nervous breakdown?"
"Did either of your parents (parent substitutes) have heart conditions?"
"Mother wants to run her children's lives. When you were growing up, did you ever feel that way too?"
"My parents are always proud of their children. When you were growing up, did you ever feel that way too?"
"Mother does not understand me. When you were growing up, did you ever feel that way too?"
"My parents often don't practice what they preach. When you were growing up, did you ever feel that way too?"
"Father wants to run his children's lives. When you were growing up, did you ever feel that way too?"
All in all, in your opinion, what one person do you take after most in character (personality, temperament, etc.)?" (This item was scored to indicate if a Midtowner reported having taken after *only the opposite sex* parent.)

Scores on this index range from 7 to 18, with low scores indicating high levels of parental adequacy, and high scores indicating low levels of parental adequacy (unfavorable), with a mean of 12 and a standard deviation of 2.

Parental Adequacy as Breadwinners
(Context of Childhood Functioning)

We measured the extent to which the Midtowners experienced their parents as functioning well or poorly outside of the household by combining the following items from the 1954 study with one from the 1974 study:

Midtowners were asked to identify "the chief problems or troubles that your parents (or parent substitute) had to face while you were growing up (ages 6–18)." This item was scored to indicate if a Midtowner reported that "unemployment, work, and/or financial" problems were "chief problems" for his parents.

"During the years you were growing up (ages 6–18), did your parents (those who brought you up) ever have a hard time making ends meet?"

"During those years you were growing up (ages 6–18), did your mother (or parent substitute) work outside the home?"

In 1974 the Midtowners were asked "When you were 13–17 years old, were your parents considered by others as wealthy, comfortably fixed, getting by, barely getting by, or poor?"

Scores on this measure range from 2 to 16, with the former indicating the highest level of parental adequacy as breadwinners (favorable) and the latter indicating the lowest level of parental adequacy (unfavorable). The index's mean is 6.6 with a standard deviation of 2.8.

Family-Kin Networks (Context of Childhood Functioning)

To measure the available social support system the Midtowners had in their pre-adult years, we used the following data from the 1954 interview:

"When you were growing up (6–18 years old), were there any other relatives (uncles, aunts, grandparents, etc.) who lived in your home with you?"

"When you were growing up (6–18 years old), were there any other relatives you were close with? How many families were you close with?"

"Did you always live with both your real parents up to the time you were 16 years old?"

The number of siblings the Midtowner reported was used in this measure.

Scores on this index range from 2 (most complete family-kin network) to 16 (least complete family-kin network) with a mean of 7 and a standard deviation of 2.5.

Pre-Adult Well-Being

The intent of this index was to globally measure symptom formation in childhood, in a manner consistent with the Rennie grades of symptom formation described in chapter 1. This global measure aggregates three domains of functioning:

a. *Intrapsychic Malfunctioning* is the sum of the Midtowners' Childhood Fear Score and Childhood Neurotic Score. As described in Langner and Michael (1963: 500) the Childhood Fear Score is measured by these 1954 interview items:

"As a child how much were you afraid of strangers? [Not At All, A Little, Much]"

"As a child, how much were you afraid of thunderstorms?"

"As a child, how much were you afraid of being left alone?"

"As a child, how much were you afraid of being on high places?"

"As a child, how much were you afraid of large animals?"

"As a child, how much were you afraid of being laughed at by other children?"

"As a child, how much were you afraid of family quarrels?"

"As a child, how much were you afraid of getting bawled out?"

The Childhood Neurotic Score comprises three 1954 items (Langner and Michael 1963: 499):

"As a child, did you fairly often have trouble falling asleep?"

"As a child, did you ever have trouble with stuttering or stammering in your speech?"

"As a child, did you fairly often have an upset stomach?"

b. *Social Malfunctioning in Childhood* is measured by the following 1954 interview items:

"I am happy only when I am at home. When you were growing up, did you ever feel that way too?"

"Some children like school; others don't. As a child, how did you feel about going to school? Would you say you liked school: very much, liked it all right, disliked it, or hated it?"

"Now as to when you were a teenager, say 13–18 years old, in those years, did you usually have dates with girls (boys) more often or less often than most other boys (girls) your age?"

Also included is the following 1974 interview item:

"When you were about 13–17 years old, did you learn to depend mainly on yourself to get things done or did you depend mainly on others to help you get things done?"

c. *Somatic Malfunctioning in Childhood* is measured by aggregating two indices. First, Midtowners' reports in 1954 of having had the following disorders before the age of 20 were summed: arthritis, asthma, bladder trouble, colitis, diabetes, hay fever, high blood pressure, sciatica or neuralgia, stomach ulcer, and/or a skin condition. Second, two 1954 interview items and one 1974 interview item were combined. The 1954 items were:

"Now, about your health in early childhood—that is, in the first six years of life: As far as you can remember or have been told, was your health in early childhood good, fair, or poor?"

"As a child, did you catch cold very often?"

From the 1974 interview, the Midtowners were asked if they had a "serious illness as a child or teenager."

We combined these three measures using the path analytic approach described by Hauser and Goldberger (1971). By definition the mean score is 0 and the standard deviation 1.[5]

Pre-1954 Level of Severity of Somatic Disorders

The 1974 interview extensively questioned the Midtowners about their somatic disorders. By using the findings of a psychophysical study of physician's ratings of the seriousness of these disorders done by Wyler et al. (1968, 1970) we were able to form measures which expressed in one number the total Severity of Somatic Disorders our respondents had up to 1954 (the present topic of discussion), as well as the total Severity of Somatic Disorders they had between 1954 and 1964, and the total Severity of Somatic Disorders they had between 1964 and 1974. Although the 1974 interview reports of somatic disorders may overlap to some extent with reports in the above measures, our Midtowners in 1974 were recalling their somatic disorders up to 1954 in the context of an adulthood of contact with physicians, mass media as well as literature presentations on aspects of physical health disorders and treatment, and their own physical health status as adults: All these factors would, we think, serve to focus our Midtowners on those somatic disorders, up to 1954, which had the most importance for their adult functioning. We should remember, however, that these are the subjective reports of our Midtowners, rather than the physical health history and examination findings of physicians. For the purpose of exploring the basic propositions of MHIM2 the reports of the Midtowners will suffice.

These are the 1974 interview items:

"I am going to read you different ailments that doctors find in their patients. Some of these are physical problems and some are emotional problems, but all can be treated by medical doctors. Please tell me whether or not you have ever had each condition I read to you. Did you ever have…(IF RESPONDENT SAYS "NOT SURE", ASK: Did a doctor ever say you had (CONDITION)?…How old were you when you or your doctor first noticed it? (RECORD AGE)." The list includes the following somatic disorders:

"Arthritis or rheumatism: stiff, painful, or swollen joints"

"Asthma: noisy and heavy breathing"

"Bladder trouble"

"Colitis: diarrhea with blood"

"Diabetes: sugar disease"

"High blood pressure"

"Stomach ulcer: stomach pains several hours after meals and during the night usually relieved by food or bicarbonate of soda"

"Chronic bronchitis: persistent coughing to bring up mucus"

"Emphysema"

"Glaucoma"

"Cataracts"

"Kidney trouble"

"Chronic liver disease (SPECIFY KIND)"

"Hardening of the arteries"

"ASK OF MEN ONLY: Prostate trouble"

"ASK OF WOMEN ONLY: Chronic, that is, long-term menstrual trouble: trouble with your periods."

A number of additional questions were asked in 1974:

"Did you ever have a stroke? How old were you [when had most recent stroke, stroke before that, stroke before that]?"

"Did you ever have a heart attack? How old were you [when had most recent heart attack, heart attack before that, heart attack before that]?"

"Do you now have any other kind of heart condition? At about what age did it start?"

"Do you now have any kind of allergy? What kind? At about what age did it start?"

"Did you ever have cancer? How old were you when it was diagnosed?"

"How many times have you had (other) major surgery? What kind of surgery did you [most recent surgery, surgery before that, surgery before that]? How old were you at the time?"

"Did you ever have any other major health problems that we haven't mentioned? What problem was that? About how old were you when you or your doctor first noticed it?"

One way to condense all of this data into one number is simply to ask the respondent this question, which was asked in about the same way in both the 1954 and 1974 interviews:

"About your health now, would you say it is: excellent, good, fair, or poor?"

This self-rated health item, however, was an important predictor of the level of mental health which the two study psychiatrist raters evaluated our Midtowners as having in 1954. Therefore it is subsumed into our measures of global mental health status in 1954 and in 1974. So rather than having the Midtowners summarize the somatic conditions data themselves, we needed some way to combine this data into one measure. Those means were provided by Wyler et al. (1968, 1970), who ingeniously developed a system for rating types of somatic disorders by their "seriousness."

We decided to use Wyler et al.'s findings to measure the relative severity of the somatic disorders reported by our Midtowners in 1974. In other words we gave the disorders *weights*, by which they were multiplied, to reflect their relative severity. In this manner we collapsed many individual indicators into one overall dimension, with the Midtown respondents having relative positions on that dimension.[6] Here are some examples of somatic disorders reported by our Midtowners and their weights:

Common cold (Head cold)	8	Asthma	78
Diarrhea (Colitis)	26	Arthritis	90
Painful menstruation		Peptic Ulcer	
(Chronic Menstrual Trouble)	37	(Stomach Ulcer)	91
Hay fever (Allergies)	43	Liver Disease	107
Overweight (Obese)	65	Heart Attack	120
Kidney infection		Bleeding in the Brain (Stroke)	123
(Kidney Trouble)	75	Cancer	125

Our Midtowners of course reported a variety of somatic disorders not on the list. Rather than rely on medical textbooks to guess-timate what their ranking would have been, we decided to give them the average weight of 63 (one half of 126). To facilitate interpretation of the sum of the weighted somatic disorders for each Midtowner, we divided it by 63, to yield the number of standard severity units that each Midtowner had up to 1954.[7] The average number of severity units up to 1954 for the total sample is 1.6 with a standard deviation of 1.8 severity units. The distribution of severity units was as follows: Of our 695 Midtowners, 212 had zero severity units up to 1954, 135 had between 0.3 and 1 severity units, 172 had between 1 and 2 severity units, and 176 had from 2 to 10 severity units.[8]

To further test the basic propositions of MHIM2, these early life experiences become predictors in our model of adult mental health status. To understand the manner in which they may predict MH, however, we need to understand the manner in which they are predicted by both the Midtowners' Sociodemographic Background characteristics and antecedent aspects of early life experiences. We turn now to the path analyses which will provide this information.

Sociodemographic Predictors of Contexts of Childhood Functioning

Body Damage. We begin with the data for path analysis, associations as measured by Pearson correlations.[9] Among all of the Midtowners, their level of Body Damage does not significantly correlate with their Age level, Gender, or their level of Socioeconomic Status of the Family of Origin (Parental SES). This is also the case in the women. But in the men the Midtowners' level of Body Damage is significantly correlated with both their Age level and Parental SES:

- There is a trend for the younger men to have higher levels of Body Damage than the older Men.
- There is also a trend for men with more favorable levels of Parental SES to have higher levels of Body Damage.

The path analysis of level of Body Damage in among all Midtowners demonstrates a significant Age and Sex interaction prediction: The predictions of Body Damage by Age level are Gender-specific. We find Age level predicts Body Damage only in the men, with the other Sociodemographic predictors controlled.

Parental Intrafamily Functioning. Among the Midtowners, both Genders combined, the Midtowners' level of Parental Intrafamily Functioning does not correlate with Gender or Parental SES. However Age level and Parental Intrafamily Functioning are correlated: There is a trend for the younger Midtowners to have more unfavorable levels of Parental Intrafamily Functioning than the older Midtowners. Among the women, neither association is statistically significant whereas among the men the trend is found.

The predictions by Sociodemographic Background characteristics of Parental Intrafamily Functioning yield a trend for the younger Midtowners to have less favorable levels of Parental Intrafamily Functioning than the older Midtowners, with the other sociodemographic predictors controlled. Note that the path analysis does not indicate that the prediction of Parental Intrafamily Functioning by Age level is Gender-specific. Although the correlation is not statistically significant in the women, it is in the same direction as in the men and of an appreciable magnitude.

Parental Breadwinner Adequacy. The Midtowners' level of Parental Breadwinner Adequacy is moderately associated in the total sample with their level of Parental SES: the more favorable their level of Parental SES, the more favorable is their level of Parental Breadwinner Adequacy. This is as anticipated: Parental Breadwinner Adequacy represents the subjective sense of economic security and well-being which the Midtowners' recall having experienced in their childhood. However the association is only of medium size, so that there are both a substantial group of Midtowners whose objectively relatively favorable Parental

SES is experienced in terms of socioeconomic disadvantage, and a substantial group whose objectively relatively unfavorable Parental SES is experienced as either an average level of socioeconomic advantage or as less unfavorable than the objective level of Parental SES might suggest. Neither Age level nor Gender are significantly correlated with Parental Breadwinner Adequacy in the total sample. The sole association, of moderate size, of Parental Breadwinner Adequacy with Parental SES is found both among the women and the men.

It comes as somewhat of a discovery, therefore, that the path analysis of Parental Breadwinner Adequacy yields two significant predictions:

• The older the Midtowners, the more favorable is their level of Parental Breadwinner Adequacy. When the Depression began (1929) many of the older Midtowners were past childhood (15–34) whereas all of the younger were children (5–14).
• The more favorable the level of the Socioeconomic Status of their Families of Origin, the more favorable is their Parental Breadwinner Adequacy.

Family-Kin Network. In the total sample, the Midtowners' level of extensivity of their Family-Kin Network in childhood is significantly correlated with both their Age level and the level of Socioeconomic Status of their Family of Origin (Parental SES):

• There is a trend for the older Midtowners to have less extensive levels of Family-Kin Network than the younger Midtowners.
• There is also a trend for Midtowners with more favorable levels of Parental SES to have more extensive levels of Family-Kin Network than Midtowners with less favorable Parental SES.

The Genders do not statistically significantly differ in their average levels of extensivity of Family-Kin Network. Among both the women and the men the associations with Age and Parental SES are statistically significant. Both Age and Parental SES significantly predict Family-Kin Network in the same manner as indicated by their correlations.

Gender-Specific Predictions of the Contexts of Childhood Functioning by Age Level and Socioeconomic Status of the Family of Origin

Among the women, neither Age nor Parental SES predict either their levels of Body Damage or Parental Intrafamily Functioning. Both Age and Parental SES predict their levels of Family-Kin Network extensivity and Parental Breadwinner Adequacy as they do among Midtowners in general.

Among the men, in contrast, all four Contexts are predicted by at least one Sociodemographic Background characteristic each: Their levels of Body Damage, Parental Intrafamily Functioning and extensivity of Family-Kin Networks are predicted by their Age level, whereas their levels of Parental Breadwinner Adequacy and Family-Kin Network extensivity are predicted by the level of Socioeconomic Status of their Family of origin. Of the four Contexts, only Family-Kin Network is not predicted in a Gender-specific manner.

Predictions of Pre-Adult Well-Being by Sociodemographic Background Characteristics and the Contexts of Childhood Functioning

We now come to a point where some aspects of our Midtowners' early life experience may be interpreted as predictors of other aspects of their early personal history. Both Pre-Adult Well-Being and the four Contexts of Childhood Functioning are measures of aspects of those experiences. They are antecedent to adult mental health status, and intervene between the Sociodemographic Background predictors and adult mental health status (and other measures of 1954 Adult Functioning). But the four Contexts of Childhood also clearly are antecedent to Pre-Adult Well-Being, and therefore intervene between the Sociodemographic Background predictors and Pre-Adult Well-Being. This follows not from the temporal sequence of data collection—most of these measures are from the 1954 interview—but from our model of the adult life cycle, derived from the basic propositions of MHIM2 and based upon our understanding of individual biological, psychological, and social development.

In the total sample we observe some significant associations involving our Midtowners' level of Pre-Adult Well-Being:

- There is a trend for Midtowners with more favorable levels of Parental SES to have more favorable levels of Pre-Adult Well-Being than those with less favorable Parental SES.
- The more favorable their level of Parental Intrafamily Functioning, the more favorable is their level of Pre-Adult Well-Being, a moderate association.
- There is also a trend for Midtowners with more favorable levels of Parental Breadwinner Adequacy to have more favorable levels of Pre-Adult Well-Being than Midtowners with less favorable Parental Breadwinner Adequacy.

The other correlations are not statistically significant.

Among the women, the associations with Parental SES, Parental Intrafamily Functioning, and Parental Breadwinner Adequacy are the only ones to be statistically significant whereas among the men only those with Parental Intrafamily Functioning and Parental Breadwinner Adequacy are statistically significant.

We next look at the predictions from our path analysis of Pre-Adult Well-Being controlling for antecedent and concurrent predictors (AC). Note that when all of the Sociodemographic Background predictors are mutually controlled, no prediction is made of Pre-Adult Well-Being either by Age overall or on a Gender-specific basis (Age and Sex interaction). The sole prediction is that the more favorable was the Midtowners' level of Parental SES, the more favorable is their level of Pre-Adult Well-Being. Then the four Contexts predictors are introduced. Two predict Pre-Adult Well-Being with the Sociodemographic Background characteristics controlled:

• The more favorable the Midtowners' level of Parental Intrafamily Functioning, the more favorable is their level of Pre-Adult Well-Being (a medium-size prediction).
• The more favorable the Midtowners' level of Parental Breadwinner Adequacy, the more favorable is their level of Pre-Adult Well-Being (a small-size prediction).

With intervening and concurrent predictors controlled (IC) the model makes the following predictions:

• Without any controls except for each other as concurrent predictors, the same two Contexts predict Pre-Adult Well-Being, specifically Parental Intrafamily Functioning and Parental Breadwinner Adequacy.
• With the Contexts controlled, of the three Sociodemographic predictors only Parental SES significantly predicts Pre-Adult Well-Being.

The predictions made by the model with all predictors mutually controlled (AIC) are as follows: Parental SES, Parental Intrafamily Functioning, and Parental Breadwinner Adequacy discretely predict Pre-Adult Well-Being net of each other and the other predictors.

Gender-Specific Predictions of Pre-Adult Well-Being by Sociodemographic Background Characteristics and the Contexts of Childhood Functioning

Among the women, the AC solution of the model yields significant predictions by Parental SES and Parental Intrafamily Functioning, in the same direction as in the total sample, whereas Parental Breadwinner Adequacy does not predict Pre-Adult Well-Being in the women. The IC solution in the women appears about equivalent to that in the total sample. With all predictors controlled, Parental SES and Parental Intrafamily Functioning predict Pre-Adult Well-Being in the women as they do in Midtowners in general, but Parental Breadwinner Adequacy does not.

The AC solution of the model in the men has different results: Only Parental Intrafamily Functioning predicts Pre-Adult Well-Being, while in the women Parental SES also predicts Pre-Adult Well-Being. The model's IC and AIC solutions yields the same results. Therefore we conclude that the prediction of Pre-Adult Well-Being by Parental SES is specific to the women.

Predictions of Level of Severity of Somatic Disorders up to 1954 by Sociodemographic Background, Contexts of Childhood Functioning, and Pre-Adult Well-Being

In the panel only two associations involving level of Severity of Somatic Disorders up to 1954 (DIS54) are observed:

- As expected, older Midtowners have higher levels of DIS54.
- There is also a trend for Midtowners with more favorable levels of Pre-Adult Well-Being to have lower levels of DIS54.

Neither Gender, Parental SES, nor the four Contexts, are statistically significantly correlated with DIS54.

The women's level of DIS54 is however statistically significantly correlated with four other characteristics:

- There is a trend for the older women to have higher levels of Severity than the younger women.
- There is a trend for women with more unfavorable levels of Body Damage to have higher levels of DIS54 than women with less unfavorable levels of Body Damage.
- There is a trend for women with more unfavorable levels of Parental Intrafamily Functioning to have higher levels of DIS54.
- There is a trend for women with more unfavorable levels of Pre-Adult Well-Being to have higher levels of DIS54.

In sharp contrast, among the men, only Age level is statistically correlated with DIS54: There is a trend for the older men to have higher levels of Severity than the younger men.

Among Midtowners in general, the path analysis yields the following predictions when each predictor is controlled for antecedent and concurrent predictors (AC):

- The older the Midtowners, the higher is their level of DIS54.
- The more unfavorable their level of Body Damage, the higher is their level of DIS54.
- The more unfavorable their level of Pre-Adult Well-Being, the higher is their level of DIS54.

When each predictor is controlled for intervening and concurrent predictors (IC), two predictions are made by the model:

- The more unfavorable their level of Pre-Adult Well-Being, the higher is their level of DIS54.
- The older the Midtowners, the higher is their level of Severity, with the other Sociodemographics, the Contexts, and Pre-Adult Well-Being controlled.

When all predictors are controlled for each other (AIC), only one prediction is made: The more favorable the Midtowners' level of Pre-Adult Well-Being, the lower is their level of Severity of Somatic Disorders up to 1954.

Gender-Specific Predictions of Level of Severity of Somatic Disorders up to 1954 by Sociodemographic Background, Contexts of Childhood Functioning, and Pre-Adult Well-Being

Among the women, the AC solution of the path model yields four predictions:

- The older the women, the higher is their level of DIS54. This is also the case among Midtowners in general.
- The less favorable their levels of Body Damage and Parental Intrafamily Functioning, the higher is their level of DIS54. The prediction by Body Damage is also seen among Midtowners overall, but not that by Parental Intrafamily Functioning.
- The less favorable is their level of Pre-Adult Well-Being, the less favorable is their level of DIS54. This is also the case among Midtowners in general.

When the IC solution of the path model in the women is reviewed, one predictor in addition to those found among Midtowners in general, Age and Pre-Adult Well-Being, is found—Body Damage. In the AIC solution of the path model in the women, Age, Body Damage and Pre-

Adult Well-Being discretely predict DIS54 net of the other predictors and each other, whereas in the total sample only Pre-Adult Well-Being was statistically significant.

The AC solution of the path model in the men displays the following predictions:

- As in the women, Age and Pre-Adult Well-Being predict DIS54.
- Only in the men does Family-Kin Network predict DIS54: The more extensive the men's Family-Kin Network in childhood, the higher is their level of DIS54.

The IC solution of the path model in the men yields the following findings:

- As in the women, Age predicts DIS54.
- Whereas Pre-Adult Well-Being predicts DIS54 in the women, it does not in the men.
- More extensive Family-Kin Networks and more favorable levels of Parental Intrafamily Functioning both predict higher levels of Severity in the men, but not in the women. Level of Body Damage does not predict DIS54 in the men although it does in the women.

With these differences in the AC and IC solutions of the path models between the Genders, it is interesting to observe that in the AIC solution in each Gender two out of the three statistically significant predictors of DIS54 are the same, namely Age and Pre-Adult Well-Being. Whereas only in the men is Family-Kin Network discretely significant, only in the women is Body Damage discretely significant. We conclude that these two Contexts of Childhood Functioning make Gender-specific predictions of DIS54.

Summary and Conclusions

In this chapter we have progressed in our exploration of the basic propositions of MHIM2 by enriching our models of the Midtowners' lives with two sets of measures of early life experience, the four Contexts of Childhood and Pre-Adult Well-Being, which is an overlay of the Midtowners' levels of Intrapsychic, Somatic and Social Functioning before adulthood. In addition we have introduced a global measure of their physical health history before 1954, that is their level of Severity of Somatic Disorders up to 1954, which weights the physical health diagnoses which our Midtowners either received from doctors, parents or other family members, or from themselves according to the "seriousness ranks" developed by Wyler et al. (1968, 1970). We have seen that predictions made of our Midtowners' levels of these measures by antecedent predictors are as often Gender-specific—statistically significant and substantial in only one Gender—as they are found in both Genders to a statistically significant extent. In view of the extensive research literature on differences between the Genders this might not be surprising, although many if not most of the particular differences and similarities observed here could not have been anticipated before the analyses were actually computed.

Equipped with a half-dozen measures measuring significant biopsychosocial characteristics of the Midtowners' lives prior to 1954, we may now proceed to test the basic propositions of MHIM2 with respect to predicting the Midtowners' adult mental health status.

Notes

1. Confer the following additional references on the modern understanding of the biopsychosocial approach: Morse 1979; Phillips et al. 1987; Rodin and Voshart 1986; Sperry 1975; and Stein et al. 1987.
2. See appendix 5.1.
3. Two comprehensive reviews for the interested reader are as follows: Anderson et al. (1979) and Bradburn et al. (1979). Of particular interest is Brewin et al. (1993: 94), which demonstrates that "...the data on personal memories that are available from naturalistic studies suggest that psychiatric patients' recall is as reliable as that of nonpatients. What can be said with more confidence is that recall of significant past events does not appear to be affected by mood state." Also of great interest are van IJzendoorn (1995) and Fox (1995).
4. An early study of the implications of Body Damage for adult functioning was presented by Landis and Bolles (1942), interesting because it was representative of the type of biopsychosocial research and theory in this area which undoubtedly influenced the design of the Midtown Study in 1954.
5. Statistically sophisticated readers will find a detailed presentation in the Statistical Appendices.
6. Also collected in 1974 were ratings by our Midtowners as to the extent to which their lives were effected by the somatic disorders, ranging from "trouble it gives you now" to "aftereffects," depending upon the type of somatic disorder. We decided to give these impairment ratings the overall label of "Seriousness" and thus we termed the somatic disorders with the Wyler et al. weights as "Severity of Somatic Disorders." "Seriousness" data is not reported here.
7. We caution that the Midtown Longitudinal Study is *not* a source of normative information about these predictors of adult mental health. Some other approaches to measuring global physical health status are discussed in the following references (among many): Garrity et al. 1978; Hunt et al. 1981; Read et al. 1987; Schliefer et al. 1985; and Schwab et al. 1978.
8. The severity of history of somatic disorders is an operationalization of the now open-ended DSM-IV Axis III (Physical Health Disorders relevant to mental

health). The advantage of so operationalizing Axis III is demonstrated in D'Ercole et al. (1991).

9. We shall describe the correlation between two variables in the present tense, as no model is being applied to their association.

Appendix 5.1

To understand the ways in which MHIM2 is a unique longitudinal study, in terms of its community sample and its measures of pre-adult experience in a social psychiatric epidemiological context, consult the following references to some outstanding longitudinal studies which have been examined by the authors: Thomas and Chess (1984); Costa and McCrae (1980); studies presented in Erlenmeyer-Kimling and Miller (1986); Berkeley et al. (1987); Pinsky et al. (1987); Spitzer (1987); Stallones (1987); Vaillant and Vaillant (1981, 1990); Cui and Vaillant (1987); Long and Vaillant (1984); Phillips et al. (1987); Vaillant (1979); Vaillant and Schnurr (1988); Aldwin et al. (1989); Werner (1989); Shedler and Block (1990); and Murphy et al. (1991).

The junior author offers the following comments about some of these references:

1. Vaillant and Schnurr (1988) use data from the Harvard Alumnae Study to demonstrate that the global functioning Axis V of DSM-III-R (which references the year up to the time of diagnosis) delineates persons in need of mental health treatment just as well as syndromal approaches defined by diagnostic criteria.

2. Costa and McCrae (1980) use data from the longitudinal Normative Aging Study to demonstrate that Positive Affect (satisfaction with life) and Negative Affect (dissatisfaction with life) predict such aspects of subjective well-being as happiness. Yet Positive Affect has distinctively different psychological health predictors than does Negative Affect! They point out (1980: 675) that their "data effectively rule(s) out the alternative explanation that associations between happiness and personality result solely from the mediating effect of temporary moods or states. This finding is also impressive as indirect evidence of the enduring effects of these dimensions of personality."

3. Murphy (1986) reviews three true longitudinal studies (the present study, the Lundby Study 1947–1972, and the Stirling County Longitudinal Study) and one pseudolongitudinal study, i.e., repeated cross-sectional samples over time from the same population, namely the Survey Research Center's National Sample Study, United States 1957–1976 (Veroff et al., 1981), concluding (1986: 113) that "more women than men at mid-century were found to have experienced depression and/or anxiety. By the end of the quarter, women and men in a few to several age groups were more equal in this regard than they had been earlier. In each study, (an) interpretation was offered to the effect that social and historical changes may have contributed to these epidemiologic trends...it is suggested that the findings deserve attention as generating hypotheses for further research."

4. In a recent publication from the classic Stirling County study, Murphy et al. (1991) establish that residents of that community of low socioeconomic status were vulnerable to incurring depression and anxiety, as defined by criteria closely resembling DSM-III, as well as continuing to be depressed and/or anxious over the study period if they were ill at baseline.

5. Spitzer (1987) is notable in his careful questioning of the value of longitudinal studies as an exploratory methodology, which is of course the nature of the study reported in this monograph. (His subject was a proposal to extend the classic Framingham study [Dawber 1980] into a more general study of aging.) Thus his point of view should be stated in his own words (1987: 181–82):

> Now a basic question is: When do you do a cohort study? To the credit of the persons reporting the first of these two works, the analysis was done on a historical cohort, going back into the past and coming to the present, with all the advantages that strategy implies in follow-up time, cost, and so forth. Nevertheless, the approach still implies fairly heavy costs and methodological difficulties, as well as bias in the follow-up—both expected and detectable, and unsuspected. It seems

to me that if you are going to use up finite resources in health services or clinical research—resources that are expended in large sums in a relatively short period of time for either randomized controlled trials or cohort studies, controlled or otherwise, historical or concurrent—then you really have to have a strong hunch about what you are pursuing.

MHIM2 demonstrates how an exploratory longitudinal study exploring the "hunches" of its fundamental theorem and basic propositions can yield important leads to health researchers regarding how adult health status develops from early childhood on, within various sociodemographic and historical settings.

References

Aldwin, Carolyn M., Avron Spiro, Michael R. Levenson, and Raymond Bossé. "Longitudinal findings from the Normative Aging study: I. Does mental health change with age?" *Psychology and Aging* 4 (September 1989): 295–306.

Anderson, Ronald, Judith Kasper, Martin R. Frankel, and Associates. 1979. *Total Survey Error*. San Francisco: Jossey-Bass, Inc.

Berkeley, Janet L., Ilana Israel, and Joseph Stokes. "Health assessment in the Framingham Offspring Study: a research proposal." *Journal of Chronic Disease* 40 (1987 suppl. 1): 169S–76S.

Bradburn, Norman M., Seymour Sudman, and Associates. 1979. *Improving Interview Method and Questionnaire Design*. San Francisco: Jossey-Bass, Inc.

Brewin, Chris R., Bernice Andrews, and Ian H. Gotlib. "Psychopathology and early experience: a reappraisal of retrospective reports." *Psychological Bulletin* 113 (January 1993): 82–98.

Costa, Paul T. and Robert R. McCrae. "Influence of extraversion and neuroticism on subjective well-being: happy and unhappy people." *Journal of Personality and Social Psychology* 38 (April 1980): 668–78.

Cui, Xing-jia and George E. Vaillant. "Antecedents and consequences of negative life events in adulthood: a longitudinal study." *American Journal of Psychiatry* 152 (January 1996): 21–26.

D'Ercole, Ann, Andrew E. Skodal, Elmer Struening, James L. Curtis, and Joel Millman. "Diagnosis of Physical Illness in Psychiatric Patients Using Axis III and a Standardized Medical History." *Hospital & Community Psychiatry* 42 (April 1991): 395–99.

Dawber, Thomas R. 1980. *The Framingham Study: The Epidemiology of Atherosclerotic Disease*. Cambridge, MA: A Commonwealth Fund Book, Harvard University Press.

Erlenmeyer-Kimling, L. and Nancy E. Miller. 1986. *Life-Span Research on the Prediction of Psychopathology*. Hillsdale, NJ: Lawrence Erlbaum Associates.

Fischer, Anita K., Janos Marton, Ernest J. Millman, and Leo Srole. 1979. "Long-range influences on adult mental health: The Midtown Manhattan Longitudinal Study, 1954–1974," in *Research in Community and Mental Health, Vol. 1*, edited by Roberta G. Simmons, 305–33. Greenwich, CT: JAI Press.

Fox, Nathan A. "Of the way we were: Adult memories about attachment experiences and their role in determining infant-parent relationships: A commentary on van Ijzendoorn (1995)." *Psychological Bulletin* 117 (May 1995): 404–10.

Garrity, Thomas F., Grant W. Somes, and Martin B. Marx. "Factors influencing self-assessment of health." *Social Science & Medicine* 12 (March 1978): 77–81.

Hauser, Robert M. and Arthur S. Goldberger. 1971. "The Treatment of Unobservable Variables in Path Analysis," in *Sociological Methodology 1971*, edited by Herbert L. Costner, 81–117. San Francisco: Jossey-Bass, Inc.

Hunt, Sonja M., S. P. McKenna, J. McEwen, Jan Williams, and Evelyn Papp. "The Nottingham Health Profile: subjective health status and medical considerations." *Social Science and Medicine* 15A (May 1981): 221–29.

Landis, Carney and Majorie Bolles. 1942. *Personality and Sexuality of the Physically Handicapped Woman.* New York: Paul B. Hoeber, Inc., Medical Book Department of Harper & Brothers.

Langner, Thomas S. and Stanley T. Michael. 1963. *Life Stress and Mental Health: The Midtown Manhattan Study.* Glencoe, IL: The Free Press.

Long, Jancis V. and George E. Vaillant. "Natural history of male psychological health, XI: escape from the underclass." *American Journal of Psychiatry* 141 (March 1984): 341–46.

Morse, Richard B. "Estimating reciprocal effects between psychological distress and perceived health status." Paper presented to the NYS Sociological Association, October 19–20, 1979.

Murphy, Jane M. "Trends in depression and anxiety: men and women." *Acta Psychiatrica Scandinavia* 73 (February 1986): 113–27.

Murphy, Jane M., Donald C. Olivier, Richard R. Monson, Arthur M. Sobol, Elizabeth B. Federman, and Alexander H. Leighton. "Depression and anxiety in relation to social status." *Archives of General Psychiatry* 48 (March 1991): 223–28.

Phillips, Katherine W., George E. Vaillant, and Paula Schnurr. "Some physiologic antecedents of adult mental health." *American Journal of Psychiatry* 144 (August 1987): 1009–13.

Pinsky, Joan L., Paul E. Leaverton, and Joseph Stokes. "Predictors of good function: the Framingham study." *Journal of Chronic Disease* 40 (1987 suppl. 1): 159S–67S.

Read, J. Leighton, Robert J. Quinn, and Martha A. Hoefer. "Measuring overall health: an evaluation of three important approaches." *Journal of Chronic Diseases* 40 (1987 suppl. 1):7S–21S.

Rodin, Gary, and Karen Voshart. "Depression in the medically ill: an overview." *American Journal of Psychiatry* 143 (June 1986): 696–705.

Schliefer, Steven J., Steven E. Keller, Samuel G. Siris, Kenneth L. Davis, and Marvin Stein. "Depression and immunity: lymphocyte function in ambulatory depressed patients, hospitalized schizophrenic patients, and patients hospitalized for herniorrhaphy." *Archives of General Psychiatry* 42 (February 1985): 129–33.

Schwab, John J., Neal D. Traven and George J. Warheit. "Relationships between physical and mental illness." *Psychosomatics* 19 (August 1978): 458–63.

Shedler, Jonathan and Jack Block. "Adolescent drug use and psychological health: a longitudinal inquiry." *American Psychologist* 45 (May 1990): 612–30.

Sperry, Roger W. "Mental phenomena as causal determinants in brain functions." *Process Studies* 5 (Winter 1975): 247–56.

Spitzer, Walter O. "Commentary: Predictors of good function: the Framingham Heart Study and health assessment in the Framingham Offspring/Spouse Study." *Journal of Chronic Diseases* 40 (1987 Suppl 1): 181S–82S.

Srole, Leo. "Social integration and certain correlaries: an exploratory study." *American Sociological Review* 21 (December 1956): 709–16.

Stallones, Reul A. "Epidemiological studies of health: a commentary on the Framingham studies." *Journal of Chronic Diseases* 40 (1987 suppl. 1): 177S–80S.

Stein, Marvin, Steven J. Schleifer, and Steven E. Keller. 1987. "Psychoimmunology in clinical psychiatry," in *Annual Review of Psychiatry/Volume 6,* edited by Robert E. Hales and Allen J. Frances, 210–34. Washington, DC: American Psychiatric Association.

Thomas, Alexander and Stella Chess. "Genesis and evolution of behavioral disorders: From infancy to early adult life." *American Journal of Psychiatry* 141 (January 1984): 1–9.

Vaillant, George E. "Natural History of Male Psychologic Health: Effects of Mental Health on Physical Health." *New England Journal of Medicine* 301 (December 1979): 1249–54.

———. 1983. *The Natural History of Alcoholism.* Cambridge, MA: Harvard University Press.

Vaillant, George E. and Paula Schnurr. "What is a case? A 45-year study of psychiatric impairment of a college sample selected for mental health." *Archives of General Psychiatry* 45 (April 1988): 313–19.

Vaillant, George E. and Caroline O. Vaillant. "Natural History of Male Psychological Health X: Work as a Predictor of Positive Mental Health." *American Journal of Psychiatry* 138 (November 1981): 1433–40.

———. "Natural History of Male Psychological Health, XII: A 45-Year Study of Predictors of Successful Aging at Age 65." *American Journal of Psychiatry* 147 (January 1990): 31–37.

Van IJzendoorn, Marinus H. "Adult attachment representations, parental responsiveness, and infant attachment: A meta-analysis on the predictive validity of the Adult Attachment Interview." *Psychological Bulletin* 117 (May 1995): 387–403.

Veroff, Joseph, Elizabeth Douvan, and Richard A. Kulka. 1981. *The inner American: a self-portrayal from 1957 to 1976.* New York: Basic Books.

Werner, Emmy E. "High-risk children in young adulthood: a longitudinal study from birth to 32 years." *American Journal of Orthopsychiatry* 59 (January 1989): 72–81.

Wyler, Allen R., Minoru Masuda, and Thomas H. Holmes. "The Seriousness of Illness rating scale." *Journal of Psychosomatic Research* 11 (December 1968): 363–74.

———. "The Seriousness of Illness rating scale: reproducibility." *Journal of Psychosomatic Research* 14 (March 1970): 59–64.

6

The Midtown Longitudinal Study Panel's Mental Health from 1954 to 1974

The objectives of this chapter are:

1. To detail the distribution of the Midtowners' adult mental health status in 1954 and in 1974.
2. To detail the Gender-specific Generational difference in adult mental health status of the women versus the men at age 40–59.
3. To present the predictions made by our model of the adult life cycle, derived from the basic propositions of MHIM2, of the Midtowners' level of Mental Health in 1954, both in the total panel (Genders combined) and in each Gender separately.
4. To broaden our model of the adult life cycle with (1) three new measures of 1954 Adult Functioning (Affective Symptoms, Excess Intake, and Social Network Density) while (2) also reintroducing 1954 Mental Health and 1954 Socioeconomic Status (SES) as predictors of 1974 Mental Health, and (3) introducing four measures of 1954 to 1974 Developments (Mental Health Treatment, Affective Episodes, Increase in Level of Severity of Somatic Disorders from 1954 to 1964, and Increase in Level of Severity of Somatic Disorders from 1964 to 1974). All of these are derived from the basic propositions of MHIM2.
5. To present the predictions made by our enriched life-span model of the Midtowners' level of Mental Health in 1974, both in the total sample (Genders combined) and in each Gender separately.
6. To present the predictions made by our model of the adult life cycle of Generation- and Gender-specific Mental Health, to determine the extent to which our biopsychosocial predictors explain this phenomenon.

* * *

We have accomplished the following preparatory tasks up to this point:

1. We have become familiar with the use of path analysis to test some the basic propositions of MHIM2 involving simple and corrected predictions

111

of the Midtowners' Own SES in 1954 and their level of Mental Health in 1954 and 1974.

2. We have seen the limited extent to which adult mental health status in 1954 and in 1974 may be predicted from such predictors as Sociodemographic Background characteristics, and, when appropriate, level of Mental Health in 1954 and level of SES in 1954.

3. We have become acquainted with six measures of the early life experiences and pre-1954 life experiences of the Midtowners, including the four Contexts of Childhood Functioning, Pre-Adult Well-Being, and Severity of Somatic Disorders up to 1954. These are needed to fully explore the basic propositions of MHIM2.

4. We have learned to what extent these six measures may be predicted from Sociodemographic Background characteristics and, as appropriate, their antecedent measures of the Midtowners' pre-1954 life experiences.

We now proceed to further explore the basic propositions of MHIM2 by determining how much we may increase the predicted percentage of the Midtowners' adult mental statuses. Our model of adult mental health status will be further enriched with four additional measures of the Midtowners' pertinent life experiences between 1954 and 1974. We shall determine the extent to which the model explains the finding that the adult mental health status of our Later Midtown women at age 40–59 is more favorable than that of our Earlier women while no change is discernible among our Midtown men. In so doing we explore the premise introduced in chapter 1 that the association of social age and adult mental health in women might be predicted by their pre-adult circumstances, that is, the era and milieu of their childhood and adolescence.

The Mental Health of the Women and the Men after Twenty Years of Aging

An important epidemiological concern is the possibility that a pattern of change or stability in adult mental health status might be Gender-specific. To explore this possibility tables 6.1 and 6.2 present the crosstabulations of global mental health in 1954 versus 1974 for the Younger and Older women, whereas tables 6.3 and 6.4 present those crosstabulations for the Younger and Older men. They bear examining in some detail.

Older Women (40–59 in 1954; 60–79 in 1974). When we examine table 6.1 we see that the Older women whose 1954 mental health was Moderate show the most change, specifically to either Mild or Impaired, with 28 (55 percent) displaying favorable change and 11 (22

TABLE 6.1
The Global Mental Health of the Older Women in 1974 versus 1954

1974: 1954:		Well	Mild	Moderate	Impaired	Total
Well	n	22+	11	2–	2–	37
	row %	59.5	29.7	5.4	5.4	17.9
	column %	50.0	13.3	4.3	5.9	
Mild	n	14	37+	17	4–	72
	row %	19.4	51.4	23.6	5.6	34.8
	column %	31.8	44.6	37.0	11.8	
Moderate	n	6–	22	12	11	51
	row %	11.8	43.1	23.5	21.6	24.6
	column %	13.6	26.5	26.1	32.4	
Impaired	n	2–	13–	15	17+	47
	row %	4.3	27.7	31.9	36.2	22.7
	column %	4.5	15.7	32.6	50.0	
Total	n	44	83	46	34	207
	%	21.3	40.1	22.2	16.4	100.0

The Older Women were 60–79 in 1974.
+ and – indicate that the observed count of subjects having particular levels of global mental health in 1954 and 1974 was either greater than or less than the count expected by chance alone.
Pearson Chi Square with 9 df = 65.97, p < .000005
Pearson Correlation = 0.48
Kappa = 0.21

percent) unfavorable change. But the three other levels of 1954 mental health are stable, so that the number of Older women having Well, Mild, or Impaired mental health in 1954 and again in 1974 is well above the level expected by chance alone.[1]

Younger Women (20–39 in 1954; 40–59 in 1974). The Younger women who had a mild level of Mental Health in 1954 strongly tend to change by 1974, 29 percent to a more favorable level (scoring Well), and 29 percent to a less favorable level (scoring Moderate or Impaired) (see table 6.2). As with the Older women the other three levels of 1954 mental health are stable, so that the numbers of Later women displaying Well, Moderate, or Impaired MH in 1954 and again 1974 are greater than those expected by chance alone.

Older Men (40–59 in 1954; 60–79 in 1974). When we look at table 6.3, we see first that the fraction of Impaired Older men in 1954 and

TABLE 6.2
The Global Mental Health of the Younger Women in 1974 versus 1954

1974:		Well	Mild	Moderate	Impaired	Total
1954:						
Well	n	27+	20	3–	1–	51
	row %	52.9	39.2	5.9	2.0	26.2
	column %	50.0	27.4	6.1	5.3	
Mild	n	24	34	21	3–	82
	row %	29.3	41.5	25.6	3.7	42.1
	column %	44.4	46.6	42.9	15.8	
Moderate	n	2–	14	19+	6	41
	row %	4.9	34.1	46.3	14.6	21.0
	column %	3.7	19.2	38.8	31.6	
Impaired	n	1–	5	6	9+	21
	row %	4.8	23.8	28.6	42.9	10.8
	column %	1.9	6.8	12.2	47.4	
Total	n	54	73	49	19	195
	%	27.7	37.4	25.1	9.7	100.0

The Younger Women are 40–59 in 1974.
+ and – indicate that the observed count of subjects having particular levels of global mental health in 1954 and 1974 was either greater than or less than the count expected by chance alone.
Pearson Chi Square with 9 df = 70.96, p < .000005
Pearson Correlation = 0.53
Kappa = 0.23

1974 is the same (11 percent), while a small gain of 3 percent is shown for the fraction Well. But when we look within the table we see that their MH tended to be stable if it was Well or Impaired in 1954, and unstable if it was Mild or Moderate in 1954. Only those who were Well or Impaired in 1954 are more likely to again score at the same level in 1974 than predicted by chance alone. The Older men who had Mild MH in 1954 shift either favorably to Well (24 percent) or unfavorably to Moderate or Impaired (22 percent), whereas the Older men who had Moderate MH in 1954 tend to change, either favorably to Well or Mild (64 percent) or unfavorably to Impaired (21 percent). In fact, statistical analysis shows that the fraction of the Older men who were Moderate in 1954 and Impaired in 1974 is disproportionately large; clinically the MH of these men was the most precarious.

Younger Men (20–39 in 1954; 40–59 in 1974). The Younger men display about the same patterns of global mental health (as seen in

TABLE 6.3
The Global Mental Health of the Older Men in 1974 versus 1954

1974: 1954:		Well	Mild	Moderate	Impaired	Total
Well	n	10+	15	0–	1	26
	row %	38.5	57.7	0	3.8	20.6
	column %	33.3	24.2	0	7.1	
Mild	n	14	31	12	1	58
	row %	24.1	53.4	20.7	1.7	46.0
	column %	46.7	50.0	60.0	7.1	
Moderate	n	4	14	4	6+	28
	row %	14.3	50.0	14.3	21.4	22.2
	column %	13.3	22.6	20.0	42.9	
Impaired	n	2	2–	4	6+	14
	row %	14.3	14.3	28.6	42.9	11.1
	column %	6.7	3.2	20.0	42.9	
Total	n	30	62	20	14	126
	%	23.8	49.2	15.9	11.1	100.0

The Older Men were age 60–79 in 1974.
+ and – indicate that the observed count of subjects having particular levels of global mental health in 1954 and 1974 was either greater than or less than the count expected by chance alone.
Pearson Chi Square with 9 df = 35.67, $p < .00005$
Pearson Correlation = 0.42
Kappa = 0.12

table 6.4) as did the Younger women (as seen in table 6.2). Midtowners who score in the Well, Moderate, and Impaired ranges of 1954 mental health tend to again score in the same range in 1974, while those who score in the Mild level in 1954 are the least likely to score in that range again in 1974.

Generation-Separated Cohort Global Mental Health and Gender

As the senior author puzzled over the lack of a clinically appreciable difference in the global mental health of the panel over twenty years of adult aging, a scientific controversy was developing over how statistical findings allegedly concerning "aging" are to be understood, that is, how to interpret statistical differences in individual characteristics which are found to change with "age." This controversy specifically addressed the difficulties, if not impossibilities, of distinguishing

TABLE 6.4
The Global Mental Health of the Younger Men in 1974 versus 1954

1974: 1954:		Well	Mild	Moderate	Impaired	Total
Well	n	17+	17	4	0–	38
	row %	44.7	44.7	10.5	0	22.8
	column %	37.0	23.0	12.5	0	
Mild	n	25	39	13	7	84
	row %	29.8	46.4	15.5	8.3	50.3
	column %	54.3	52.7	40.6	46.7	
Moderate	n	3–	10	13+	2	28
	row %	10.7	35.7	46.4	7.1	16.8
	column %	6.5	13.5	40.6	13.3	
Impaired	n	1–	8	2	6+	17
	row %	5.9	47.1	11.8	35.3	10.2
	column %	2.2	10.8	6.3	40.0	
Total	n	46	74	32	15	167
	%	27.5	44.3	19.2	9.0	100.0

The Younger Men were age 40–59 in 1974.
+ and – indicate that the observed count of subjects having particular levels of global mental health in 1954 and 1974 was either greater than or less than the count expected by chance alone.
Pearson Chi Square with 9 df = 40.67, p < .00001
Pearson Correlation = 0.38
Kappa = 0.18

among the statistical effects of Age, Generation, and Period on individual characteristics:

1. "Age" effects refer to how people change as they move from one stage of the life cycle to the next stage. These effects are the subject of psychosocial studies by such scholars as Levinson et al. (1978) and Davitz and Davitz (1980), among others; and of the best-selling journalism of Sheehy (1995). In this study "Age" means *biological age.*

2. "Generation" refers to the experiences shared by people who were born in the same era. For example, those Midtowners who were aged 40–59 in 1954[2] were born between 1895 and 1914, before World War I. This Earlier Generation of Midtowners experienced their adolescent years (age 12–16) between 1907 and 1934, a period spanning World War I and the beginning of the Great Depression. In contrast those Midtowners who were aged 40–59 in 1974 were born between 1915

and 1934, during or after World War I and up to the beginning of the Great Depression. They experienced adolescence between 1927 and 1954, a period including the Great Depression, World War II, and the Korean conflict. The Midtowners within each of these two Generations may resemble each other in certain ways and differ from people born in other eras simply because they shared certain experiences due to the historical context of their life course. At any one time people born in different eras may be measured and compared statistically. The findings may be attributed to the fact that people born in different eras were in different stages of their life cycle when studied (i.e., in terms of Age effects). But this interpretation would be incorrect if, in fact, the measurements were of personal characteristics caused by the historical context of their lives (Generation rather than Age effects)[3].

This very important concept may be expressed as follows: membership in a Generation defines the *social age* of the members.

3. "Period" effects take place when there is change in the meaning of a measurement performed in two different eras on the same people. For example, in this study the Midtowners were asked both in 1954 and in 1974 whether they had ever had a nervous breakdown. If that term had not been defined as part of the question ("did you ever have a period of a week or more during which you could not perform your normal activities?"), but had been left to the Midtowners to define for themselves, then a "Period" effect might have occurred. Specifically, as a result of such an error (which did not in fact happen), in 1954 the semantic meaning of the phrase "nervous breakdown" might have differed from that in 1974, perhaps as a result of the purported psychologizing of American society (Veroff et al. 1981). Then no statistical finding from a comparison of the distribution of responses to this item in 1954 with those in 1974 could be interpreted except in terms of semantic drifts over twenty years. Such a finding might be of interest to lexicographers, but not to mental health practitioners and researchers.

As we studied and reflected upon this new approach to "age" we came to realize that our expectation that the mental health of the Midtowners would change unfavorably to a statistically significant extent with the passage of twenty years had not considered the circumstance that Midtowners of various (biological) age levels had been born in different historical eras, and thus had shared different historical experiences in different social, economic, political, and cultural contexts (i.e., were of different levels of social age). These circumstances might have been completely different contexts for the adult life cycle of our

Midtowners. We then found a way to untie the gordian knot of Age, Period, and (Decade of Birth) Generation effects on an individual characteristic, assuming that the essential meaning of that individual characteristic had not changed between 1954 and 1974 (the two periods of measurement in MHIM2):

1. Each Midtowner was of age 40–59 in one of the two periods, either in 1954 or in 1974.

2. If our assumption is valid then (a) associations with levels of biological age can be measured by comparing the item's distributions in 1954 and 1974; and (b) associations with levels of social age can be measured by comparing the item's distribution when the Midtowners are age 40–59, specifically by comparing the 1954 measurement for the Earlier Generation with the 1974 measurement for the Later Generation.

During the course of developing the global mental health measure, Midtown Longitudinal Study researchers established that the measure and its component items had equivalent socioclinical correlates in 1954 and 1974, and therefore that the 1974 measure was a true replication of the 1954 measure; thus the possibility of Period effects was ruled out. Then we could proceed with our Age and Generation analysis of global mental health.

The results to be presented may be previewed as follows: Srole and Fischer (1980) found a consistent Generation effect by comparing the adult mental health status of the Earlier and the Later Generations. When they repeated this comparison for each Gender separately a most unexpected finding emerged: Only the women show a Generation effect, with the Later Generation having more favorable levels of mental health than the Earlier Generation.[4] This Gender-specific Generation effect, observed uniquely in MHIM2, is an epidemiological finding which has powerfully driven us to further exploration using the model derived from the basic propositions of this study.

Gender and the Global Mental Health of the Generations

We have already shown how, by pairing the 1954 measurement of the Earlier Midtowners with the 1974 measurement of the Later Midtowners, when the measurement was obtained in both 1954 and 1974, we obtain a set of measurements of the entire panel at age 40–59, which can be statistically analyzed to estimate a Generation effect. Now we shall pair the 1954 MH of the Earlier Midtowners with the

TABLE 6.5
Cohort Mental Health Impairment in the Women by Generation

		Later 40–59 in 74	Earlier 40–59 in 54	Total
Impaired	n	19–	47+	66
	row %	28.8	71.2	16.4
	column %	9.7	22.7	
Not Impaired	n	176+	160–	336
	row %	52.4	47.6	83.6
	column %	90.3	77.3	
Total	n	195	207	402
	%	48.5	51.5	100.0

+ and – indicate that the observed count of subjects having particular levels of global mental health in 1954 and 1974 was either greater than or less than the count expected by chance alone.
Pearson Chi Square with 1 df = 12.29, p < .0005
Pearson Chi Square with Continuity Correction = 11.37, p < .001
Pearson Correlation = 0.17
Relative Risk (Odds Ratio) = 2.72, 95% confidence interval 1.53 to 4.83

TABLE 6.6
Cohort Mental Health Impairment in the Men by Generation

		Later 40–59 in 74	Earlier 40–59 in 54	Total
Impaired	n	15	14	29
	row %	51.7	48.3	9.9
	column %	9.0	11.1	
Not Impaired	n	152	112	264
	row %	57.6	42.4	90.1
	column %	91.0	88.9	
Total	n	167	126	293
	%	57.0	43.0	100.0

+ and – indicate that the observed count of subjects having particular levels of global mental health in 1954 and 1974 was either greater than or less than the count expected by chance alone.
Pearson Chi Square with 1 df = 0.36, p = 0.546
Pearson Chi Square with Continuity Correction = 0.17, p = 0.68
Pearson Correlation = 0.04
Relative Risk (Odds Ratio) = 1.27, 95% confidence interval 0.59 to 2.73

TABLE 6.7
Cohort Mental Health Wellness in the Women by Generation

		Later 40–59 in 74	Earlier 40–59 in 54	Total
Well	n	54+	37–	91
	row %	59.3	40.7	22.6
	column %	27.7	17.9	
Not Well	n	141–	170+	311
	row %	45.3	54.7	77.4
	column %	72.3	82.1	
Total	n	195	207	402
	%	48.5	51.5	100.0

+ and – indicate that the observed count of subjects having particular levels of global mental health in 1954 and 1974 was either greater than or less than the count expected by chance alone.
Pearson Chi Square with 1 df = 5.53, p = .019
Pearson Chi Square with Continuity Correction = 4.98, p = .026
Pearson Correlation = -0.12
Relative Risk (Odds Ratio) = 0.57, 95% confidence interval 0.35 to 0.91

TABLE 6.8
Cohort Mental Health Wellness in the Men by Generation

		Later 40–59 in 74	Earlier 40–59 in 54	Total
Well	n	46	26	72
	row %	63.9	36.1	24.6
	column %	27.5	20.6	
Not Well	n	121	100	221
	row %	54.8	45.2	75.4
	column %	72.5	79.4	
Total	n	167	126	293
	%	57.0	43.0	100.0

Pearson Chi Square with 1 df = 1.85, p = .174
Pearson Chi Square with Continuity Correction = 1.50, p = .221
Pearson Correlation = -0.08
Relative Risk (Odds Ratio) = 0.68, 95% confidence interval 0.39 to 1.18

1974 MH of the Later Midtowners, to measure the MH of each Generation at age 40–59. Specifically, this measure characterizes each member of the Panel by the global mental health level he or she had at age 40–59, whether in 1954 (for the Earlier Generation Midtowners) or in 1974 (for the Later Generation Midtowners).[5] Although of the same biological age level, the members are thus characterized by their social age, as members of the Earlier or the Later Generation. We shall focus specifically on the two most clinically meaningful levels of cohort global mental health, Well and Impaired. Tables 6.5 and 6.6 present the distribution of Mental Health Impairment of women and men at age 40–59, and tables 6.7 and 6.8 that of Mental Health Wellness of women and men at age 40–59.

Earlier Midtown women are almost three times more likely to have impaired mental health at age 40–59 than the Later women (see table 6.5). Of the Earlier women, 23 percent are impaired at that age, as compared with only 10 percent of the Later women. But there is no such trend among the Midtown men (see table 6.6): only 11 percent of the Earlier men are impaired, in contrast to 9 percent of the Later men.

Conversely, when we examine the results for cohort mental health wellness presented in table 6.7 we find that Later Midtown women are almost twice as likely as Earlier women to be well. Of the Later women, 28 percent are well at age 40–59, as compared with only 18 percent of the Earlier women. No such trend emerges among the men, as shown in table 6.8. Of the Later men 28 percent are well (the same level as among women) whereas 21 percent of the Earlier men are well.

These findings lead us to wonder about possible historical changes in the biopsychosocial antecedents of mental health of the Midtown women between the Earlier and Later Generations, which might be associated with a favorable change in the Midtown women's aggregate level of mental health. The Midtown men of different Generations may also have had historical changes in the antecedents of their mental health, but, if so, these changes did not produce an overall difference in the rate of Impaired MH between men of different Generations. Specifying the nature of these differences in antecedents, to the greatest extent that our data allows us, is a logical step in the exploration of the basic propositions of MHIM2; and may be viewed also as a psychohistorical challenge (Simonton 1990). To specify these differences, we first study the biological, social, and psychological antecedents of adult global mental health.

Biopsychosocial Models of Global Mental Health

In 1979 we presented our initial biopsychosocial models (Fischer et al. 1979). The selection of variables was based on our theoretical thinking about the etiology of adult global mental health at that time. It was there that the historical element became especially prominent in the Midtown Longitudinal Study, with the first publication of the finding for Generations and Mental Health.

We now begin with our final model of the Midtowners' mental health status at baseline, in 1954.

Predictions of 1954 Mental Health Status by Sociodemographic Background, Contexts of Childhood Functioning, Pre-Adult Well-Being, and Severity of Somatic Disorders up to 1954

We have already established a baseline for how little the 1954 mental health status of the Midtowners can be explained by sociodemographic predictors alone—five percent. All of the additional predictors are studied in retrospect; that is, when the Midtowners had already attained their level of global mental health in 1954 they were asked to recall various aspects of their life history. Recall also that the data on Somatic Disorders up to 1954 was collected in the 1974 interview, which took a far more extensive and detailed physical health history from the Midtowners than had been obtained in 1954.[6]

Consistent with the basic proposition of MHIM1, the Midtowners' level of Mental Health 1954 is correlated with all of the predictors with the sole exception of extensivity of Family-Kin Networks. The predictions of our life-span model of 1954 Mental Health, with Intervening and Concurrent predictors controlled (IC), are as follows:

1. Pre-1954 Somatic Disorders were mostly experienced in adolescence and early adulthood (before 1954). The Midtowners' level of severity of these disorders has a low predictive relationship with 1954 Mental Health.
2. The level of Pre-Adult Well-Being, net of Pre-1954 Somatic Disorders, moderately predicts the 1954 level of Mental Health.
3. Of the four Contexts of Childhood Functioning indices, only Body Damage does not have a low predictive association with global mental health net of the other Contexts, Pre-Adult Well-Being, and Pre-1954 Somatic Disorders.[7] The prediction for level of extensivity of Family-Kin Network controlling intervening and concurrent variables is more than its statistically insignificant correlation would have lead us to expect. We have already learned in chapter 5 that in both the women and the men, Family-Kin Network is predicted by both level of biological age (hence-

forth simply "Age") and Parental Socioeconomic Status (SES). But now we discover that Family-Kin Network's role as a predictor of MH54 is also a result of its concurrent associations with the other three Childhood Contexts, specifically Parental Breadwinner Adequacy, Parental Intrafamily Functioning, and Parental Breadwinner Adequacy.

4. The Sociodemographic Background predictors are introduced in two steps. First Sex, Age level, and Parental SES are entered. Parental SES has a low predictive association with mental health status separate from the other Sociodemographic Background predictors, Contexts, Pre-Adult Well-Being, and Pre-1954 Somatic Disorders.

Then the Sex by Age Interaction is introduced. We again find, in a different statistical venue, an association among the Midtown women, between being Older (40–59 in 1954 rather than 20–39 in 1954) and less favorable average levels of 1954 mental health, as compared to the Younger women, to a greater extent than would be explained by the associations of Age (i.e., being Older) and Sex (i.e., being women) simply added together.

The finding for Parental SES is notable precisely because the other predictors do not function as intervening variables to fully explain its association with 1954 mental health status, an issue highlighted by the basic propositions of MHIM2. Parental Breadwinner Adequacy summarizes the recalled experience of favorable or unfavorable Parental SES from an adult perspective in both our women and men. The Midtowners' levels of extensivity of Family-Kin Network are also predicted in both Genders by Parental SES. We have also found that in the women the more favorable was the level of Parental SES the more favorable is their level of Pre-Adult Well-Being; this was not the case in the men. Finally in neither Gender does the Midtowners' level of Parental SES predict their level of Severity of Somatic Disorders up to 1954.

Thus this finding suggests that the impact of Parental SES on adult mental health is quite broad and diffuse. This substantiates the basic proposition of MHIM1 and is consistent with the public health literature on the possible status of socioeconomic status as a "fundamental cause" of disease (Link and Phelan 1995) cited in chapter 3.

Yet another aspect of this finding is particularly noteworthy: Although all of the other predictor variables were controlled, the Age-by-Sex interaction was predictive, so that this interaction was also not explained away by the intervening predictors.

The second solution of our model controls each predictor variable for concurrent and antecedent variables (AC). The findings are as follows:

1. The Midtowners' level of Parental SES makes a low prediction of MH54. When the Age-by-Sex interaction is introduced, it is predictive and again suggests that Older women have a less favorable average level of 1954

global mental health than can be explained by the added associations of Age and Sex alone.

2. When the Contexts of Childhood are introduced, again three out of four have low predictive associations with global mental health in 1954, net of each other and the demographic variables. But this time it is Body Damage that has a low association, and Family-Kin Network that does not.[8]

3. Pre-Adult Well-Being has a moderate predictive association with 1954 global mental health net of the Contexts of Childhood Functioning and the Sociodemographic Background predictors.

4. Pre-1954 Somatic Disorders does not predict 1954 mental health status when Pre-Adult Well-Being, Contexts of Childhood Functioning, and Demographic Variables are controlled. It is thus "explained away" by its associations with the antecedent predictors, particularly by those with Age level, Body Damage, and Pre-Adult Well-Being in the women and with Age level, Family-Kin Network, and Pre-Adult Well-Being in the men.

The third solution of our model, which controls each predictor for its associations with all other predictors (AIC), finds five predictors of MH54 net of their associations with all of the other predictors, specifically the Midtowners' levels of Parental SES, Age level in the women rather than in the men (the interaction prediction), Parental Breadwinner Adequacy, Parental Intrafamily Functioning, and Pre-Adult Well-Being.

In summary, adult mental health status in 1954 is associated with and predicted by the following predictors with any and all path model controls: the Age-by-Sex interaction, Parental SES, Parental Breadwinner Adequacy, Parental Intrafamily Functioning, and Pre-Adult Well-Being. Family-Kin Network extensivity predicts 1954 MH when intervening predictors are controlled, even though overall it was not associated with MH54. The level of somatic disease history up to 1954 is associated with MH54 but does not predict MH54 when antecedent predictors are controlled. These findings substantiate the basic proposition of MHIM1, by demonstrating differences in the mental health composition of subgroups of Midtowners with varying biopsychosocial background characteristics. A basic proposition of MHIM2, that there will be differences among subgroups of Midtowners of different biological age levels and genders, is also substantiated.

Predictions in Each Gender of 1954 Mental Health Status

We begin with the associations between MH54 and the model predictors in each Gender. In the women all of the predictors are associated with MH54 whereas in the men only four are associated: Parental

SES, Parental Intrafamily Functioning, Parental Breadwinner Adequacy, and Pre-Adult Well-Being. Thus only in the women and not in the men do Age level, Body Damage, Family-Kin Network, and Severity of Somatic Disorders up to 1954 correlate with MH54.

Our model for women with antecedent and concurrent predictors controlled (AC) makes the following predictions: The younger the women were, the more favorable is their average level of MH54. The more favorable was their Parental SES level, the more favorable is their level of MH54. The more favorable was their level of Parental Intrafamily Functioning, the more favorable is their MH54 level. The more favorable was their level of Pre-Adult Well-Being, the more favorable is their level of MH54.

The predictions of our model in the women with intervening and concurrent predictors (IC) controlled are, first, that the higher the level of Severity of Somatic Disorders up to 1954 the women experienced, the less favorable is their 1954 level of Mental Health. Then again the more favorable were their levels of first Pre-Adult Well-Being and then Parental Intrafamily Functioning, the more favorable is their level of MH54. Finally, the Younger women have a more favorable average level of MH54 than do the Older women.

The finding that Parental SES is no longer predictive of MH54 is quite notable: all of its predictive power is explained by its associations with intervening and concurrent predictors. It is also notable that Parental Breadwinner Adequacy, the subjective representation of Parental SES, also does not predict MH54 when intervening and concurrent predictors are controlled.

With all predictors in the women controlled for all other predictors (AIC), the model predicts the following: the Younger women have a more favorable average level of Mental Health in 1954 than do the Older women. The more favorable were their levels of first Parental Intrafamily Functioning and then Pre-Adult Well-Being, the more favorable is their level of MH54.

In the men the model with antecedent and concurrent predictors controlled (AC) predicts the following: as was the case in the women, the more favorable was the men's level of Parental SES, the more favorable is their 1954 level of Mental Health. Unlike in the women, the men's level of Age does not predict their level of MH54. Then again as in the case of the women the more favorable were the men's levels of first Parental Intrafamily Functioning and then Pre-Adult Well-Being, the more favorable is their level of MH54.

The predictions of the model in the men with intervening and concurrent predictors controlled (IC) are as follows: unlike the case in the women, their level of Severity of Somatic Disorders up to 1954 does not predict their MH54. The more favorable was their level of Pre-Adult Well-Being, the more favorable is their MH54, as with the women. But the rest of the model findings for men are markedly and importantly unlike those for women: (1) Parental Intrafamily Functioning level is *not* predictive of the men's MH54 with the intervening predictors controlled; (2) the more favorable was the men's level of Parental SES, the more favorable is their 1954 level of Mental Health; and (3) the men's level of Age does not predict their level of MH54.

With all predictors in the men controlled for all other predictors (AIC), the model predicts the following: The more favorable were their levels of Pre-Adult Well-Being the more favorable is their level of MH54. The more favorable was the men's level of Parental SES, the more favorable is their 1954 level of Mental Health. Unlike the case in the women, the men's levels of Age and Parental Intrafamily Functioning do not predict their 1954 mental health status.

The most striking difference in findings for the Midtown women vis-à-vis the men is that the prediction of increasingly unfavorable levels of 1954 adult mental health by increasingly unfavorable levels of parental socioeconomic status is explained away when the intervening predictors are controlled, but not when only the concurrent predictor of biological age level is controlled. In this sense, the association of Parental SES and 1954 MH is explained by our model, reflecting the basic propositions of MHIM2, among *only* the Midtown women. We will of course be watching for whether or not this gender difference persists in our models of levels of 1974 adult mental health.

1954 Adult Functioning and Post-1954 Developments: New Predictors of Adult Mental Health Status

Our models of 1974 Mental Health benefit from the prospective aspects of the Midtown Longitudinal Study, although they contain retrospective elements as well. That is to say that we can prospectively predict Mental Health in 1974 from data collected in 1954 that both concerned the Midtowners' functioning and other characteristics in 1954 and prior to 1954. In addition we can use data collected retrospectively in 1974, when the Midtowners had already attained their restudy Mental Health status, concerning events of the prior twenty years (from 1954 to 1974).

To model our Midtowners' Mental Health status in 1974, and to also model the change in Mental Health status which occurred from 1954 to 1974 we first add to our model aspects of the Midtowners' functioning as adults in 1954 which the basic propositions of MHIM2 imply will predict the Midtowners' 1974 level of Mental Health. These include, in addition to their 1954 levels of SES and MH (the predictions of which we have discussed in chapter 4) their 1954 levels of Extensivity of Social Network, Excess Intakes, and Affective Symptoms. Note that we treat the level of Severity of Somatic Disorders up to 1954 as a 1954 Adult Functioning predictor to simplify the model. We also study a variety of potential predictors from the 1974 reinterview which focused on the 1954 to 1974 period, all of which are implied by the basic propositions of MHIM2 to predict 1974 MH. We develop four measures of pertinent life cycle developments in adulthood, namely (1) whether the Midtowners had sought Mental Health Treatment between 1954 and 1974, (2) whether they had affective episodes between 1954 and 1974, (3) whether their level of Severity of Somatic Disorders increased between 1954 and 1964, and (4) whether their level of Severity of Somatic Disorders increased between 1964 and 1974.

The composition of these new predictors is as follows:

1954 Affective Symptoms. Midtowners were asked the following questions in the 1954 interview:

"Do you feel that you have had your share of good luck in life?"

"On the whole, life gives you pleasure. Do you agree or disagree?"

"Nothing ever turns out for me the way I want it to."

"Of course we all have our emotional ups and downs, and laymen as well as doctors know that these can sometimes have effects on our health. What about yourself? In general, would you say that most of the time you are in high spirits, good spirits, low spirits, or, very low spirits?" (For scoring purposes, high and good spirits were combined, as were low and very low spirits.)

The Affective Symptoms Measure scores range from 0 (no symptoms) to 4 (most symptoms), with a mean of 0.3 and a standard deviation of 0.7.

Excess Intakes in 1954. This measure counts respondents' reports in 1954 of "often" drinking more coffee, smoking more cigarettes, eating more food, and/or drinking more alcoholic beverages "than is good for you." Scores on this measure range from 0 (no excess intakes) to 4 (most excess intakes), with a mean of 1 and a standard deviation of 1.

Social Network Density in 1954.[9] This measure sums the standardized scores for respondents' reports in 1954 of how many friends, relatives, and neighbors they have, plus how many organizations in which they are active. By definition the mean is 0 and standard deviation 1.

1954 Level of Severity of Somatic Disorders. We have identified this measure in chapter 5 as the level of Severity of Somatic Disorders up to 1954. To somewhat simplify our model, we have chosen to include this measure as a 1954 Adult Functioning predictor in our models of 1974 Adult Functioning and Changes in Adult Functioning from 1954 to 1974.

Increase in Level of Severity of Somatic Disorders from 1954 to 1964. This measure is constructed in the same way as the level up to 1954, except that only those disorders which are reported by the Midtowners to have been first diagnosed or otherwise known to them between eleven and twenty years prior to the interview are included. As with the 1954 level of Severity of Somatic Disorders, this measure is expressed in standard units corresponding to a physical illness of median severity. Between 1954 and 1964 417 Midtowners (60 percent of the 695) reported no new physical health disorders at all (0 units); 101 Midtowners (14 percent) reported from 0.4 to 1 units of new disorders; 105 (15 percent) reported from 1 to 2 units of new disorders; 36 (5 percent) reported from 2 to 3 units of new disorders, and 36 (5 percent) reported from 3 to 8 units of new disorders. The mean is 0.7 units with a standard deviation of 1 unit.

Increase in Level of Severity of Somatic Disorders from 1964 to 1974. This measure is constructed in the same way as the level up to 1954, except that only those disorders which are reported by the Midtowners to have been first diagnosed or otherwise known to them between zero and ten years prior to the interview are included. No new disorders (0 units) are reported by 214 Midtowners (31 percent); from 0.4 to 1 units by 81 Midtowners (12 percent); 1 to 3 units by 226 Midtowners (32 percent); 3 to 5 units by 139 Midtowners (20 percent); and 5 to 11 units by 35 Midtowners (5 percent). The mean is 2 units with a standard deviation of 2 units.

Affective Episodes Measure. This measure of unusual affective episodes (mood swings from normal to high and/or low) includes the following 1974 interview items:

"Have there been times when you changed for a whole week or more from your usual self to unusually high spirits, i.e., everything in you seemed to be working at top speed and you felt on top of the world?"

"Have there (also) been times when you changed for a whole week or more to unusually low spirits, i.e., when you felt utterly miserable and everything seemed too much of an effort for you?"

Scores on this measure range from 0 (neither type of episode occurred), reported by 525 Midtowners (76 percent) to 2 (both types of episode occurred), reported by 31 Midtowners (4 percent), with a mean of 0.3 and a standard deviation of 0.5; thus 139 Midtowners (20 percent) reported only one type of episode, virtually all the depressive type.

Mental Health Treatment. This measure assigns a 1 to respondents who answered any of the following 1974 items in the affirmative for the period following the 1954 interview, and a 0 to the others.

"People sometimes go to a hospital or nursing home for an emotional or nervous condition. Of course, these too are medical problems treated by doctors and nurses. Have you ever been in a hospital or nursing home for such an emotional or nervous condition?"

"Have you ever gone to a hospital clinic or non-hospital clinic for an emotional or nervous condition? How old were you when you went to such a clinic for the first time?"

"To get help for an emotional problem or nervous condition people also go to other kinds of professionals outside of a hospital or clinic. For such personal problems have you ever gone to a private psychiatrist, psychologist, counselor, clergyman, social worker, group therapist, or other similar kind of professional?"

Scores on this measure ranged from 0 (no psychiatric treatment) to 1 (psychiatric treatment), with a mean of 0.2 and a standard deviation of 0.4, so that about 20 percent sought treatment.

Predictions of 1974 Mental Health Status by Sociodemographic Background, Contexts of Childhood Functioning, Pre-Adult Well-Being, 1954 Adult Functioning, and 1954–1974 Developments

Weak associations are observed between MH74 and Age level, Parental SES, Parental Intrafamily Functioning, Parental Breadwinner Adequacy, Pre-Adult Well-Being, Severity of Somatic Disorders up to 1954, Affective Symptoms in 1954, extensivity of Social Networks in 1954, SES in 1954, increase in Severity of Somatic Disorders from 1954 to 1964 and also from 1964 to 1974, Affective Episodes, and

Mental Health Treatment. A moderate correlation is found between MH74 and MH54. Only Gender, Body Damage, and extensivity of Family-Kin Network are not associated with MH74.

The path model with concurrent and intervening predictors controlled (IC) makes the following predictions:

1. Increasing levels of all four Post-1954 Developments weakly predict less favorable levels of 1974 Mental Health net of each other, specifically (1) having sought Mental Health Treatment between 1954 and 1974; (2) having had periods of unusually high or low spirits lasting at least a week between 1954 and 1974 (Affective Episodes); (3) having had somatic disorders come to their attention between 1954 and 1964; and (4) having had somatic disorders come to their attention between 1964 and 1974.

2. Of the six aspects of Baseline Adult Functioning (in 1954), three prospectively predict Mental Health in 1974 net of each other and of the Post-1954 Developments. The Midtowners' level of Mental Health in 1954 has a moderate association, whereas their level of Severity of Somatic Disorders and Own SES have low associations. Affective Symptoms, Social Network Density, and Excess Intakes do not discretely predict 1974 Mental Health.[10]

3. Pre-Adult Well-Being, Contexts of Childhood Functioning, and Demographic Variables all yield the same findings: No discrete predictions of 1974 Mental Health are made. The manifest reason for this is that they all are associated with MH54. In this sense none of the pre-1954 predictors have "sleeper effects" on MH74, that is to say, none have associations with MH74 that are not explicable by their associations with MH54.

The predictions made by the path model controlling concurrent and antecedent predictors (AC) are as follows:

1. Among the demographic variables, Age level and Parental SES predict 1974 Mental Health net of each other and Gender, at a low level.

2. Controlling for demographic variables and each other, only Parental Intrafamily Functioning predicts 1974 Mental Health, at a low level. Thus controlling for antecedent and concurrent predictors, this Context of Childhood Functioning may be a risk factor for 1974 Mental Health, although specified by its associations with intervening variables, particularly 1954 Mental Health. It is noteworthy that Midtowners whose memories in 1954 suggested that their parents had difficulty in functioning as parents are still at an elevated risk of unfavorable Mental Health twenty years later. Epidemiological research about the key impact of parents in the childhood years has continually appeared.[11]

3. Pre-Adult Well-Being makes a low prediction of 1974 Mental Health net of the Contexts of Childhood Functioning and Sociodemographic Background characteristics. This is explained by the association of Pre-Adult

Well-Being with the intervening variables in the model, particularly 1954 Mental Health and also the level of Severity of Somatic Disorders up to 1954.

4. Of the six indices of Baseline Adult Functioning, only two discretely predict 1974 Mental Health when antecedent and concurrent predictors are controlled. These are the level of Severity of Somatic Disorders up to 1954 and MH54.

5. Finally all four Post-1954 Developments make low predictions of 1974 Mental Health controlling for all other predictors, including each other.

The predictions made by the model with each predictor controlled for all other predictors are as follows:

1. Demographic Variables, Contexts of Childhood Functioning, and Pre-Adult Well-Being all have no discrete association with 1974 Mental Health.

2. Of the six Baseline Adult Functioning measures, only the level of Severity of Somatic Disorders up to 1954 and Mental Health discretely and prospectively predict 1974 Mental Health.

3. All four of the Post-1954 Developments discretely predict 1974 Mental Health.

Summary. These findings, from a model which incorporates a variety of potential biopsychosocial predictors reflecting various periods in the life cycle, strongly substantiate the basic propositions of MHIM2. Although the average mental health of the total panel of Midtowners did not change with twenty years of aging, there was a trend for the older Midtowners to have less favorable levels of mental health in 1974 than the younger Midtowners. Midtowners with increasingly unfavorable levels of Parental Socioeconomic Status (SES) had increasingly unfavorable levels of 1974 MH. Midtowners with less favorable levels of 1974 MH had memories of their parents consistent with less adequate functioning in the parental role as compared with Midtowners with more favorable levels of 1974 MH. Midtowners whose levels of well-being before adulthood were less favorable had less favorable 1974 MH as compared to Midtowners whose levels of pre-adult well-being were more favorable. Midtowners with more favorable levels of 1974 MH had more favorable levels of 1954 SES as compared with Midtowners with less favorable levels of 1974 MH. All four post-1954 developments discretely predicted 1974 MH. As a separate post-1954 development, Mental Health Treatment will receive special attention in chapter 7. With the expansion of the models, the percentage of 1954 mental health explained in the total panel of Midtowners increases from five to twenty one percent, in the women from six to twenty four percent, and in the men from one to fifteen percent. These findings strongly substantiate the basic propositions of MHIM2.

Gender-Specific Predictions of 1974 Mental Health Status

Among the Midtown women, seventeen of the eighteen predictors (all except Family-Kin Network) are associated with MH74. In the men, however, only ten of the eighteen predictors are correlated with MH74 at a level greater than expected by chance alone. These are: Parental SES, Pre-Adult Well-Being, 1954 Affective Symptoms, 1954 Social Network Density, Severity of Somatic Disorders up to 1954, 1954 SES, 1954 MH, increase in Severity of Somatic Disorders from 1964 to 1974, Affective Episodes, and Mental Health Treatment. Only in the women, and not in the men, do Age level, the four Contexts of Childhood Functioning, 1954 Excess Intakes, and increase in Severity of Somatic Disorders from 1954 to 1964 predict their MH74 level.

The predictions of MH74 in the women by our model with antecedent and concurrent predictors controlled (AC) indicate the following trends:

- The Younger Midtown women tended to have more favorable levels of 1974 MH than the Older women.
- More favorable levels of Parental SES predicted more favorable levels of MH in 1974.
- More favorable levels of Parental Intrafamily Functioning predicted more favorable levels of 1974 MH.
- More favorable levels of Pre-Adult Well-Being predicted more favorable levels of MH74.
- The more favorable their MH54 level, the more favorable is their MH74 level.
- The more unfavorable their level of Affective Episodes, the more unfavorable is their level of MH74.
- The higher the increase in their level of Severity of Somatic Disorders between 1954 and 1964, the more unfavorable is their level of MH74.
- The higher the increase in their level of Severity of Somatic Disorders between 1964 and 1974, the more unfavorable is their level of MH74.

The predictions by the model of the women's MH74 level with intervening and concurrent predictors controlled (IC) are as follows:

- The higher their level of Affective Episodes, the more unfavorable is their 1974 level of Mental Health.

- Both periods of increase in Severity of Somatic Disorders predict MH74: the higher the women's level of increase in Severity, the more unfavorable is their MH74.
- The more favorable their MH54 level, the more favorable is their MH74 level.

With each predictor controlled for the levels of all other predictors (AIC), the model predicts the women's level of 1974 Mental Health as follows:

- The more unfavorable their level of Affective Episodes, the more unfavorable is their level of MH74.
- The higher their increase in level of Severity of Somatic Disorders, the less favorable is their 1974 level of Mental Health.
- The more favorable their level of MH54, the more favorable is their level of MH74.

The predictions of MH74 in the men by our model with antecedent and concurrent predictors controlled (AC) are as follows:

- The more favorable the Parental SES level of the men, the more favorable is their MH74. Age level was not predictive among the men, although it was among the women.
- The more favorable their MH54 level, the more favorable is their MH74 level. The predictions of MH74 in the women by Parental Intrafamily Functioning and Pre-Adult Well-Being are not found in the men.
- There was a trend for the Midtown men with increasingly unfavorable levels of Somatic Disorders up to 1954 to have increasingly unfavorable levels of 1974 Mental Health.
- The higher the increase in their level of Severity of Somatic Disorders between 1964 and 1974, the more unfavorable is their level of MH74. Although the level of increase of Severity between 1954 and 1964 and the level of Affective Episodes predict the MH74 level of the women, they do not in the men.
- The men who sought treatment for mental health problems between 1954 and 1974 have a more unfavorable level, on the average, of MH74 than do those who did not seek help. This is not seen in the women.

The predictions by the model of the men's MH74 level with intervening and concurrent predictors controlled (IC) are as follows:

- The higher their level of Affective Episodes, the more unfavorable is their 1974 level of Mental Health.
- The men who sought mental health treatment had a more unfavorable level of 1974 Mental Health than those who did not seek treatment.

• The higher the men's level of increase in Severity of Somatic Disorders from 1964 to 1974 the more unfavorable is their MH74. These last two predictions are the same as those in the women. But the level of increase in Severity in the women between 1954 and 1964 also predicted their level of MH74.

• The more favorable the men's MH54 level, the more favorable is their MH74 level. This of course is seen in the women, unlike the following two predictions seen only in the men:

• The more favorable the men's level of Severity of Somatic Disorders up to 1954, the more favorable is their level of 1974 Mental Health.

• The more favorable the men's level of SES in 1954, the more favorable is their level of MH74.

With each predictor controlled for the levels of all other predictors (AIC), the model predicts the men's level of 1974 Mental Health as follows:

• Those men who sought treatment for mental health problems between 1954 and 1974 have a less favorable average level of 1974 Mental Health than did those men who did not seek help. Note that the prediction in the women made by their level of Affective Episodes is not seen in the men.

• The higher their increase in level of Severity of Somatic Disorders between 1964 and 1974, the less favorable is their 1974 level of Mental Health. This is found in the women, whose MH74 is also predicted by their level of increase in Severity between 1954 and 1964.

• The more favorable their level of MH54, the more favorable is their level of MH74. This, of course, is seen in the women, unlike the following two predictions seen only in the men:

• The more favorable the men's level of Severity of Somatic Disorders up to 1954, the more favorable is their level of 1974 Mental Health.

• The more favorable the men's level of SES in 1954, the more favorable is their level of MH74.

Summary. We add to the running comparison of the women and the men just completed that the single consistent predictor of 1974 level of Mental Health, regardless of which model is used and regardless of whether the Midtowners under study are the women, the men, or the total panel, is the 1954 level of Mental Health. Note that in the total panel neither Age nor the Age-by-Sex interaction discretely predict 1974 Mental Health. As compared with the minimal models of chapter 4, the explained percentage of 1974 levels of Mental Health increases in the total Midtown panel from 21 to 29 percent, in the women from 24 to 32 percent, and in the men from 17 to 24 percent.

Biopsychosocial Models of Generation-Separated Mental Health

Having already defined a social age-related mental health measure termed "Generation-separated Mental Health" (GMH),[12] we proceed to further explore the basic propositions of MHIM2. In so doing we use Age level to code Generation, since each Midtowner of the Earlier Generation has a constant of twenty years added to his or her age in 1954 to represent their membership in the Earlier rather than Later Generation. At the same time we control for the relative age (in a twenty-year span) of each Midtowner within his or her Generation.

We also introduce as a predictor the Generation-separated measure of level of Severity of Somatic Disorders at age 40–59, analogous to Generation-separated Mental Health. For our Earlier Generation of Midtowners this is their level of Severity up to 1954, whereas for our Later Generation this is their level of Severity up to 1974 (i.e., summing their level up to 1954, and their levels of increase from 1954 to 1964 and from 1964 to 1974). We abbreviate this predictor as GSD.

Our path analysis of GMH begins by reviewing its associations with its predictors. We observed low to medium size associations with Age, Gender, Parental SES, Body Damage, Parental Intrafamily Functioning, GSD, and Pre-Adult Well-Being.

The model of Generation-separated Mental Health (GMH) estimating paths with concurrent and intervening variables controlled (IC) obtained about the same results as for 1954 Mental Health (MH54), with one exception: Parental Breadwinner Adequacy is no longer associated with GMH as it had been with MH54. The Age-by-Sex interaction continues to be predictive with all available predictors of GMH controlled. This indicates that the statistical controls for the life-span predictors do not reduce the association of the Age-by-Sex interaction with GMH to such an extent that no prediction is made.[13]

The second set of predictions of this model of GMH, with the paths adjusted for concurrent and antecedent predictors (AC) are by and large the same findings as for MH54. The exceptions are as follows: (1) the Age-by-Sex interaction is not predictive; (2) the Midtowners' level of Body Damage does not predict their level of GMH as it had their level of MH54; (3) GSD predicts GMH. Note that the Midtowners' level of Severity up to 1954 had not predicted their level of MH54.

The predictions of the model with each predictor controlled for all other predictors (AIC) are substantially parallel to those for MH54 with the following exceptions: (1) Parental Breadwinner Adequacy is not predictive of GMH as it had been of 1954 Mental Health; and (2) GSD predicts GMH.

Gender-specific Models of Generation Mental Health

How may the predictions of GMH vary within each Gender according to the manner in which our path model is solved? Answering this question is a vital part of exploring the basic propositions of MHIM2.

We begin with the correlations in each Gender between GMH and its predictors. In the Midtown women all but two of the nine predictors are associated with GMH, namely Parental SES and Family-Kin Network. In the men only four out of the nine predictors are associated with GMH: Parental SES, Pre-Adult Well-Being, and GSD. Thus only in the women are Age, Body Damage, Parental Intrafamily Functioning, and Parental Breadwinner Adequacy associated with GMH.

The path model in the women of their level of GMH with Antecedents and Concurrents controlled (AC) yielded predictions in the expected directions by their Age level, Body Damage level, level of Parental Breadwinner Adequacy, level of Pre-Adult Well-Being, and GSD. Parental Intrafamily Functioning was not predictive.

With each predictor controlled for intervening and concurrent predictors (IC) the path model in the women of their level of GMH found predictions in the expected directions by their GSD, level of Pre-Adult Well-Being, Parental Intrafamily Functioning level, level of density of Family-Kin Network, and Age level; the latter is not reduced to statistical nonsignificance by being controlled for all other predictors in the model.

The path model in which each predictor is controlled for antecedent, intervening, and concurrent predictors (AIC) established, in the expected directions, predictions of the women's GMH by their Age level, level of Parental Intrafamily Functioning, Pre-Adult Well-Being level, and GSD.

The path model in the Midtown men of their level of GMH with Antecedents and Concurrents controlled (AC) shows that predictions in the expected directions are made by their level of Pre-Adult Well-Being and GSD, both as in the case in the women. But unlike in the women, the men's levels of Age, Body Damage, and Parental Breadwinner Adequacy do not predict their GMH. Whereas Parental SES level predicts the GMH of the men, it does not do so in the women.

With each predictor controlled for intervening and concurrent predictors (IC) the path model of GMH in the men finds predictions in the expected directions made by their GSD, level of Pre-Adult Well-Being, and level of Parental SES; the latter is not seen in the women. Observed only in the women are predictions for Parental Intrafamily Functioning level, level of density of Family-Kin Network, and Age level.[14]

The path model in which each predictor is controlled for antecedent, intervening, and concurrent predictors (AIC) found, in the expected directions, predictions of the men's GMH by their level of Parental SES, Pre-Adult Well-Being level, and GSD. These are all seen in the women, who also uniquely display a prediction by Age level.

Summary. The basic propositions of MHIM2 imply that the predictions of mental health status by biopsychosocial predictors would vary among groups of Midtowners defined by their Gender. We have just reviewed findings strongly substantiating that idea. Level of Age consistently is associated with and predictive of GMH among the Midtown women, regardless of controls, and is never associated with GMH among the men. Level of Parental SES is consistently associated with and predictive of GMH among the Midtown men, but never among the women. Although Parental Breadwinner Adequacy is associated with GMH among the men, it is never predictive of GMH, whereas among the women all four Contexts of Childhood predictors are predictive in some models of GMH. Finally, both Pre-Adult Well-Being and GSD are associated with and predictive of GMH in all models for both the Midtown women and the men. We have found that whereas the baseline models of GMH predicted only 4 percent of GMH in the women and only three percent in the men, the above models predicted 11 percent in the women and 9 percent in the men, a notable improvement in predictive power.

Models of Generation-Separated Mental Health
by Gender and Generation

The basic propositions of MHIM2 address the possibility that the associations of mental health with biopsychosocial predictors would vary among groups of Midtowners separated by Gender and Generation. Prompted by the finding that the path model of GMH in the total sample generates a Gender-by-Generation prediction, we proceed to present models for the Earlier and Later men and women separately.

The IC model of GMH in the Earlier Midtown women shows that it is predicted, respectively, by their GSD, their level of Pre-Adult Well-Being, and their level of Parental Intrafamily Functioning. The AC model finds predictions of MH by their levels of Parental SES, Parental Intrafamily Functioning, and Pre-Adult Well-Being. With all predictors controlled for all other predictors (AIC), only Parental Intrafamily Functioning and Pre-Adult Well-Being predict GMH in the Earlier women.

We may note with some interest that in the Earlier women their level of Parental SES does not predict their level of GMH (which was measured in 1954) when the concurrent and intervening predictors are controlled. Recall that in the total sample the level of MH54 was discretely predicted by the level of Parental SES even with all other predictors controlled. This is not the case in the Earlier women.

The IC model in the Later women shows that their level of GMH is predicted by their level of GSD as well as by their levels of Pre-Adult Well-Being and Parental Intrafamily Functioning. The predictions made by the AC model in the Later women show the same three predictions, even with the change in statistical controls. With all predictors mutually controlled, the AIC model yields these same predictions.

We have seen that whereas in the Earlier women the level of Parental SES predicts GMH only when the sole control is for Age level in years (ranging over a twenty-year span from 40 to 59 years), in the Later women the level of Parental SES never predicts GMH. We now proceed to the predictions made by our path model in the men.

The only IC prediction of GMH in the Earlier men is by their level of Pre-Adult Well-Being. The only AC prediction of our model is again that of their level of Pre-Adult Well-Being. It is therefore inevitable that when all predictors in the Earlier men are mutually controlled, only their level of Pre-Adult Well-Being predicts their level of MH.

Among the Later men, the IC model's predictions of GMH are as follows: their level of Parental SES predicts their level of MH even with all other predictors controlled; this is not seen in the other Midtowners. This is distinct from the case with the Earlier women, where Parental SES predicts MH only when it is not controlled for the intervening predictors. We also observe that with no intervening predictors to control, their Generation-specific level of Severity of Somatic Disorders predicts the Later men's GMH. In the Later men the AC results are as follows: There was a trend for the older men in this group to have less favorable levels of GMH than the younger men in this group. Again the Later men's levels of Parental SES and GSD predict their level of GMH. Thus with all predictors controlled only both Parental SES and GSD predict the MH of the Later men.

We may summarize our Generational findings among the men as follows: Among the Earlier men only Pre-Adult Well-Being was discretely predictive of GMH, whereas among the Later men only Parental SES and GSD were discretely predictive of GMH.

Summary

We may summarize our progress in testing the basic propositions of MHIM2 with the data for Generation-separated and Gender-separated mental health as follows: Two groups defined by their Gender and Generation have a prediction made of their Generation-specific level of Mental Health (GMH) by their level of Parental SES, the Earlier women and the Later men. The association in Earlier women becomes not predictive when the intervening predictors are controlled, whereas that in the Later men persists when all predictors are controlled.

In chapter 5 we presented an account of the implications of variations of predictors in predicting a characteristic of our Midtowners, such as their mental health status. We especially emphasized the significance of a situation in which a predictor makes a prediction when controlled for antecedent and concurrent predictors, but not for intervening predictors. In such a situation the intervening predictors possibly serve as mediators of the predictions made by the predictor under study (Shepperd 1991). Applying this methodological consideration to the current problem, we conjecture that in the Earlier women their level of Parental SES predicts their level of MH because it predicts their levels of Parental Intrafamily Functioning and Pre-Adult Well-Being. In the previous chapter we learned the following about the women: (1) Their level of Parental Intrafamily Functioning was not associated with their levels of Age or Parental SES. (2) Their level of Pre-Adult Well-Being was predicted both by their level of Parental SES and by their level of Parental Intrafamily Functioning.

In the men, in contrast, their level of Parental Intrafamily Functioning was predicted by their Age level, while their level of Pre-Adult Well-Being was predicted only by their level of Parental Intrafamily Functioning, regardless of the statistical controls applied.

In establishing these findings we have fleshed out the observation in chapter 1 concerning the roots in pre-adult years of adult mental health, while demonstrating that predictions of GMH involving Parental SES and other life cycle measures are specific to some subgroups of Midtowners defined by their Gender and Generation. These variations in predictions strongly substantiate the basic propositions of MHIM2. In the next chapter we turn our attention towards another aspect of adult mental health: predictors of mental health treatment.

Notes

1. For the statistically sophisticated reader, a full detailed description of these tables may be found in the Statistical Appendices. The descriptions reported here are based on standard techniques of analyzing such tables. All of the descriptive statistics reported in this chapter have been rounded out to promote readability. Readers demanding greater quantitative precision are asked to consult the Statistical Appendices.
2. Simonton (1990) suggests twenty years as a historically significant span of years to define a generation. Sociologists use the technical term "cohort" to refer to sets of persons sharing some characteristic, and "birth cohort" to refer to sets of persons born within the same time period. See Riley (1973, 1987).
3. See the following additional references for technical presentations of the cohort analytic method: Feinstein (1985); Feinberg and Mason (1979); Srole (1979); and Srole and Fischer (1986, 1989).
4. This was a distinctly different finding than reported in other psychiatric studies of symptoms of depression and anxiety (Klerman et al. 1985; Gershon et al. 1987). Klerman and Weissman (1991) later restricted the cohort trend in depression to cohorts born after World War II, that is, following the Midtown study.
5. We remind the reader that we refer to the Earlier and Later Midtowners as being of different Generations. They differ not in *biological* age but in *social* age. This means the same thing as saying that they are of different birth cohorts. Differences between generations measure Generation effects, that is, differences between groups defined by their social age.
6. See chapter 5 for details.
7. Since of necessity Body Damage and Pre-1954 Somatic Disorders overlapped, this control may have resulted in Body Damage's just barely missing a statistically significant level of association.
8. Body Damage has not been controlled (in this solution) for either the Midtowners' levels of Pre-Adult Well-Being or of Severity of Somatic Disorders up to 1954. In contrast, Family-Kin Network has been controlled for Parental SES, which predicts it.
9. A seminal study pertaining to the role of Social Network Density in adult mental health status is that of the Joint Commission on Mental Illness and Health (Robinson et al. 1960).
10. Note that once MH54 is included in the group of measures for which a measure is statistically controlled, the resulting prediction is a prediction of change in mental health status from 1954 to 1974. The measure's association with MH74 is statistically controlled for its association with MH54, yielding a prediction of change in mental health. The Statistical Appendices present further details on this method of measuring change, and also the findings of analyses which focus specifically on a regression measure of the change from MH54 to MH74 as the outcome measure. We do not discuss these findings in this monograph because of space limitations. It must suffice to say that no additional findings of consequence came from this approach in this study.
11. The following references are indicative of the range and pervasiveness of lasting interest about this issue: Wender 1979; Weissman et al. 1984; Keller et al. 1986;

Weissman et al. 1987; Breier et al. 1988; Kendler 1988; and Shedler and Block 1990.

12. This measure has already been described in chapter 4. We also modeled the Generation-separated Mental Health of the entire panel using only the Sociodemographic Background characteristics as predictors to establish baseline estimates of the predicted percentage of GMH.

13. Logistic regression analysis of the Impaired level of Generation-separated Mental Health presented in the Statistical Appendices demonstrates the prediction by the Age-by-Sex interaction.

14. A direct inference is that the prediction of GMH by Age level is specific to the women. Remembering that Age level encodes Generation with the added specificity of relative Age level within Generation, we conclude that this finding shows the persistence of the Generation-by-Gender interaction even with all life cycle measures controlled.

References

Breier, Alan, John R. Kelsoe, Paul D. Kirwin, Stacy A. Beller, Owen M. Wolkowitz, and David Pickar. "Early parental loss and development of adult psychopathology." *Archives of General Psychiatry* 45 (November 1988): 987–93.

Davitz, Joel R. and Lois L. Davitz. 1980. *Making It: Forty and Beyond, Surviving the Mid-Life Crisis*. San Francisco: Harper San Francisco, Division of HarperCollins Publishers, Inc.

Feinstein, Alvan R. 1985. *Clinical Epidemiology. The Architecture of Clinical Research*. Philadelphia: W.B. Saunders Co.

Fienberg, Stephen F. and William M. Mason. 1979. "Identification and estimation of age-period-cohort models in the analysis of discrete archival data," in *Sociological Methodology 1979*, edited by Karl F. Schuessler, 1–67. San Francisco: Jossey-Bass.

Fischer, Anita K., Janos Marton, Ernest J. Millman, and Leo Srole. 1979. "Long-range influences on adult mental health: The Midtown Manhattan Longitudinal Study, 1954–1974," in *Research in Community and Mental Health, vol. 1*, edited by Roberta G. Simmons, 305–33. Greenwich, CT: JAI Press.

Gershon, Elliot S., Joel E. Hamovit, Juliet J. Guroff, and John I. Nurnberger. "Birth-Cohort Changes in Manic and Depressive Disorders in Relatives of Bipolar and Schizoaffective Patients." *Archives of General Psychiatry* 44 (April 1987): 314–19.

Keller, Martin B., William R. Beardslee, David J. Dorer, Philip W. Lavori, Harriet Samuelson, and Gerald L. Klerman. "Impact of severity and chronicity of parental affective illness on adaptive functioning and psychopathology in children." *Archives of General Psychiatry* 43 (October 1986): 930–37.

Kendler, Kenneth S. "Indirect vertical cultural transmission: a model for nongenetic parental influences on the liability to psychiatric illness." *American Journal of Psychiatry* 145 (June 1988): 657–65.

Klerman, Gerald L., Philip W. Lavori, John Rice, Theodore Reich, Jean Endicott, Nancy Andreasen C., Martin B. Keller, and Robert M. Hirschfield. "Birth-cohort trends in rates of major depression among relatives of patients with affective disorder." *Archives of General Psychiatry* 42 (July 1985): 689–93.

Klerman, Gerald L. and Myrna M. Weissman. "Increasing rates of depression." *Journal of the American Medical Association* 261 (April 1989): 2229–35.

Levinson, Daniel. 1978. *The Seasons of a Man's Life*, edited by Charlotte N. Darrow, Edward B. Klein, Maria H. Levinson, and Braxton McKee. New York: Alfred A. Knopf.

Levinson, Daniel, in collaboration with Judy D. Levinson. 1996. *The Seasons of a Woman's Life*. New York: Alfred A. Knopf.

Link, Bruce G. and Jo C. Phelan. "Social conditions as fundamental causes of disease." *Journal of Health and Social Behavior* (Extra Issue 1995): 80–94.

Riley, Matilda W. "Aging and cohort succession: interpretations and misinterpretations." *Public Opinion Quarterly* 37 (Spring 1973): 35–49.

———. "On the significance of age in sociology." *American Sociological Review* 52 (February 1987): 1–14.

Robinson, Reginald, David F. DeMarche, and Mildred K. Wagle. 1960. *Community Resources in Mental Health*. New York: Basic Books.

Shedler, Jonathan and Jack Block. "Adolescent drug use and psychological health: a longitudinal inquiry." *American Psychologist* 45 (May 1990): 612–30.

Sheehy, Gail. 1995. *New Passages: Mapping Your Life Across Time*. New York: Random House.

Shepperd, James A. "Cautions in Assessing Spurious 'Moderator Effects'." *Psychological Bulletin* 110 (September 1991): 315–17.

Simonton, Dean K. 1990. *Psychology, Science, and History: An Introduction to Historiometry*. New Haven, CT: Yale University.

Srole, Leo. 1979. "Macrosocial and Microsocial Crises and Their Impact on the Midtown Manhattan Follow-up Panel," in *Stress and Mental Disorder*, edited by James E. Barrett et al., 201–12. New York: Raven Press.

Srole, Leo, and Anita K. Fischer. "The Midtown Manhattan Longitudinal Study vs. 'The Mental Paradise Lost' doctrine: a controversy joined." *Archives of General Psychiatry* 37 (February 1980): 209–21.

———. 1986. "The Midtown Manhattan Longitudinal Study: Aging, Generations, and Genders," in *Community Surveys of Psychiatric Disorders. Series in Psychosocial Epidemiology 4*, edited by Myrna M. Weissman, Jerome K. Myers, and Catherine E. Ross, 77–107. New Brunswick, NJ: Rutgers University Press.

———. "Changing lives and well-being: the Midtown Manhattan Panel Study, 1954–1976" [sic]. *Acta Psychiatrica Scandinavia* 79 (1989 suppl. 348): 35–44.

———. 1982. "Gender, generations, and well-being: the Midtown Manhattan Longitudinal Study," in *Life-Span Research on the Prediction of Psychopathology*, edited by L. Erlenmeyer-Kimling and Nancy E. Miller, eds., chapter 23. Hillsdale, NJ: Lawrence Erlbaum Associates.

Veroff, Joseph, Elizabeth Douvan and Richard A. Kulka. 1981. *The Inner American: A Self-portrayal from 1957 to 1976*. New York: Basic Books.

Weissman, Myrna M., Gammon G. Davis, Karen John, Kathleen R. Merikangas, Virginia Warner, Brigette A. Prusoff, and Diane Sholomskas. "Children of depressed parents: increased psychopathology and early onset of major depression." *Archives of General Psychiatry* 44 (October 1987): 847–53.

Weissman, Myrna M., James F. Leckman, Kathleen R. Merikangas, Gammon G. Davis, and Brigette A. Prusoff. "Depression and anxiety disorders in parents and children. Results from the Yale Family Study". *Archives of General Psychiatry* 41 (September 1984): 845–52.

Wender, Paul. 1979. "Nurture and Psychopathology: Evidence from Adoption Studies." In *Stress and Mental Disorder*, edited by James E. Barrett et al., 251–64. New York: Raven Press.

7

The Midtown Longitudinal Study
of Mental Health Treatment

In 1981 two landmark studies based upon two cross-sectional surveys of representative samples of the American adult population, one in 1957 and another in 1976, were published. The primary topics of these surveys by Joseph Veroff and colleagues were (1) mental health symptom measures and their sociodemographic correlates, and (2) attitudes and past actions with respect to mental health treatment. Although different individuals were included in the 1957 and 1976 samples, the researchers were able to infer shifts in national attitudes and behaviors with respect to mental health treatment, as well as shifts in the distribution and sociodemographic correlates of various mental health symptom measures.

The Midtown Longitudinal Study is distinct from these landmark studies because:

1. The same individuals were interviewed, both in 1954 and in 1974, permitting us to directly observe the extent to which their adult functioning status remained stable or changed, and the biopsychosocial correlates of that stability or change.
2. Rather than being restricted to mental health symptom measures, the Midtown Longitudinal Study used as its primary measure *global* mental health status. We simplify the measure here to compare those Midtowners who were probably in need of mental health treatment, the Impaired, and those Midtowners who were probably not in need of mental health treatment, the Well, with those in intermediate, equivocal need of mental health treatment, those neither Well nor Impaired.
3. We test the historical generalizability of the finding in MHIM1 that those community residents who were in most need of mental health treatment were the least likely to receive it (Srole et al. 1975). If this remained true after 1954, up to 1974, with the expansion in services associated with Medicaid, Medicare, and the community mental health movement, then the MHIM1 finding generalized to MHIM2.

Our longitudinal design affords us a unique opportunity to study the biopsychosocial origins of seeking treatment for mental health problems. Unlike the case with the Veroff et al. studies[1], we have data from twenty years before our measure (in 1974) of whether or not the Midtowners sought mental health treatment between 1954 and 1974. Furthermore we have data from the 1974 reinterview which has as its temporal locus the Midtowners' life experiences prior to 1954. By studying the ways in which our model of adult mental health status in 1974 and change in mental health status between 1954 and 1974 might predict mental health treatment, we further explore the basic propositions of MHIM2. We also present the predictors of an evaluation by the Midtowners who sought help from mental health treatment of the degree to which they were in fact helped by those services.

We have applied the same approach to this Post-1954 Development as we had to mental health, namely path analysis. Use of logistic regression allows us to describe the increase or decrease in the relative chances, or *odds*, associated with a unit change in a predictor that the Midtowners will have had treatment rather than not had treatment.

We begin with the associations between the predicted characteristic and the predictors. First we note that there is no trend towards a Gender difference among Midtowners in seeking mental health treatment. Low and stable associations are observed between the Midtowners' seeking mental health treatment (which we shall abbreviate Treatment) and their levels of Age, Parental Socioeconomic Status, Body Damage, Parental Intrafamily Functioning, Family-Kin Network, Pre-Adult Well-Being, and 1954 Socioeconomic Status.

The results for the total sample of computing the path model with each predictor controlled for concurrent and intervening predictors (IC) are as follows:

1. *Post-1954 Developments*. In the total panel, none of the other three Post-1954 Developments significantly predict seeking Treatment.[2]

2. *Baseline Adult Functioning*. Of the six measures, only Own Socioeconomic Status (SES54) predicts seeking Treatment, with the other five and the Post-1954 Developments controlled. With each step of more favorable SES54, the odds of seeking Treatment from 1954 to 1974 increase by more than 40 percent. Thus Midtowners who have High-High (level 6) SES in 1954 are almost two and a half times more likely to have sought help by 1974 than those who have Low-Low (level 1) SES in 1954.

3. *Pre-Adult Well-Being*. With Baseline Adult Functioning and Post-1954 Developments controlled, the odds that Midtowners will seek Treatment

between 1954 and 1974 rise by more than 40 percent with each additional unit of impairment in Pre-Adult Well-Being. This represents a "sleeper effect" of pre-adult functioning on post-1954 Adult Functioning (Fischer et al. 1979).

4. *Contexts of Childhood Functioning.* None of the four Contexts predict seeking treatment for mental health problems controlling for Pre-Adult Well-Being, Baseline Adult Functioning, and Post-1954 Developments.

5. *Demographic Variables.* Younger Midtowners (40–59 in 1974) are more than twice as likely to seek Treatment as Older Midtowners (60–79 in 1974) even with all other predictors controlled. This is consonant with the findings of Veroff and colleagues. The Midtowners' level of Parental SES also discretely predicts their seeking treatment for mental health problems: With each additional favorable level of Parental SES, Midtowners are more than a quarter more likely to seek treatment for mental health problems between 1954 and 1974. Neither Gender nor the interaction between Age and Sex significantly predict seeking treatment for mental health problems.

The path model of seeking Treatment with each predictor controlled for antecedent and concurrent predictors (AC):

1. *Demographic Variables.* The Age level of the Midtowners predicts their seeking Treatment, with the Older Midtowners being half as likely as the Younger Midtowners to do so. The odds of seeking Treatment increase by more than a third with each additionally favorable level of Parental SES, so that Midtowners of High-High (level 6) SES are about twice as likely as those of Low-Low (level 1) SES to have sought help by 1974.

2. *Contexts of Childhood Functioning.* Two of the four Contexts significantly predict seeking Treatment, and by the same degree: Each additional level of impairment in Parental Intrafamily Functioning and in Parental Breadwinner Adequacy predicts an increase of about a third in the chances of the Midtowners seeking Treatment between 1954 and 1974.

3. *Pre-Adult Well-Being.* Even with Contexts and Demographics controlled, Pre-Adult Well-Being significantly predicts seeking Treatment: The chances of being treated increase by almost two-fifths with each additional level of impaired functioning prior to adulthood.

4. *Baseline Adult Functioning.* With their antecedents and each other controlled, the Baseline Adult Functioning measures as a group do not predict seeking treatment for mental health problems. Own level of SES in 1954 continues to have an individual predictive relationship. The lack of predictions by either Mental Health Wellness or Impairment is remarkable.

5. *Post-1954 Developments.* With all of the other predictors controlled, these do not discretely predict seeking Treatment.

The path model of seeking Treatment between 1954 and 1974, with each predictor controlled for all other predictors (AIC) yields the following predictions:

1. *Demographic Variables.* With all other predictors controlled, the Younger Midtowners are more than twice as likely as the Older Midtowners to seek Treatment. Level of Parental SES also discretely predicts seeking Treatment, so that with each more favorable level the odds of seeking Treatment increase by about a quarter.

2. *Contexts of Childhood Functioning.* Three of the four significantly correlate with seeking Treatment, but do not discretely predict seeking treatment. On the other hand the measure without an overall association, Parental Breadwinner Adequacy, has a discretely predictive association with seeking Treatment. This prediction by the Midtowners' level of experienced childhood SES, holding constant (among other predictors) their objective level of Parental SES, is most intriguing. It indicates that at any level of Parental SES, those Midtowners who experienced that level relatively unfavorably before 1954 are more likely to seek treatment for mental health problems between 1954 and 1974, decades after their childhood, than those who experienced that level relatively favorably.

3. *Pre-Adult Well-Being.* This measure discretely predicts seeking Treatment between 1954 and 1974: With each additional unit of impairment the chances of seeking treatment rises by almost 40 percent.

4. *Baseline Adult Functioning.* Among these six measures, only the Midtowners' level of SES in 1954 discretely predicts their seeking Treatment: Midtowners of High-High SES (level 6) in 1954 are almost twice as likely as those of Low-Low SES (level 1) to seek help between 1954 and 1974.

5. *Post-1954 Developments.* None either correlate with or discretely predict seeking Treatment.

The basic propositions of MHIM2, strongly supported by the findings for mental health and Treatment, imply that the Midtown women and men sought treatment for mental health problems under different circumstances, influenced by different life historical factors. Therefore we now present the path models for the Genders separately, and compare the results.

Gender-Specific Models of Mental Health Treatment

We begin with the associations between Treatment and the model predictors. In the Midtown women seeking Treatment is associated at a low level with their levels of Age, Parental SES, Parental Intrafamily Functioning, and 1954 SES. In the men, seeking Treatment correlates at a low level with their levels of Age, Parental SES, Parental Intrafamily Functioning, Pre-Adult Well-Being, 1954 SES, Impaired Mental Health in 1954, and increase in Severity of Somatic Disorders from 1954 to 1964. All of the associations found in the women are found in the men, but only the latter show the associations involving Pre-Adult Well-Being, Impaired Mental Health in 1954, and increase in Severity of Somatic Disorders from 1954 to 1964.

Findings from the path model in the Midtown women of seeking treatment for mental health problems, with each predictor controlled for concurrent and intervening predictors (IC) are as follows:

1. *Post-1954 Developments.* None predict seeking Treatment.
2. *Baseline Adult Functioning.* Higher levels of 1954 SES predict seeking Treatment after 1954. In addition, the women who had a mental health status less favorable than Well are more than twice as likely as the others to seek Treatment, although Mental Health Impairment is not predictive.
3. *Pre-Adult Well-Being.* The women's level of Pre-Adult Well-Being predicts seeking Treatment, with the chances almost doubling with each additional unit of impairment in childhood functioning.
4. *Contexts of Childhood Functioning.* The Contexts do not predict seeking Treatment.
5. *Demographic Variables.* Neither Age level nor Parental SES predict women's seeking Treatment.

The findings in the men of solving the path model controlling for intervening and concurrent predictors (IC) are as follows:

1. *Post-1954 Developments.* Unlike the case in the women, one Post-1954 Development predicts the men's seeking Treatment: With each additional level of Severity of Somatic Disorders from 1954 to 1964, the chances of the men's seeking Treatment increases by half.
2. *Baseline Adult Functioning.* The MH Impaired men are seven times as likely as the other men to seek Treatment after 1954, whereas among the women it is those whose MH54 is less than Well who are most likely to seek Treatment.
3. *Pre-Adult Well-Being.* Unlike the case with the women, in the men there is no prediction.
4. *Contexts of Childhood Functioning.* None discretely predict seeking Treatment.
5. *Demographic Variables.* Younger men are almost five times as likely to seek Treatment as Older men, when all of the other variables in the model are controlled. A similar trend is present in the women, but simply at a less than predictive level, and therefore there is no prediction for the interaction between Age level and Gender in the total panel. Parental SES

predicts seeking Treatment in the men with all other predictors controlled, unlike in the women: With each additionally favorable level of Parental SES, the men's chances of seeking Treatment rise by two-fifths.

The path model in the women with each predictor controlled for concurrent and antecedent predictors (AC) yields the following findings:

1. *Demographic Variables.* Controlling for Parental SES, Younger women are about twice as likely to seek Treatment as Older women. Controlling for Age level, women's chances of seeking Treatment rise by almost two-fifths with each additionally favorable level of Parental SES.
2. *Contexts of Childhood Functioning.* None predict women's seeking Treatment.
3. *Pre-Adult Well-Being.* With each additional level of impairment in childhood functioning, the chances of the women seeking Treatment between 1954 and 1974 rise by two-fifths.
4. *Baseline Adult Functioning.* Only the women's 1954 level of SES discretely predicts their seeking Treatment, with the chances of women doing so increasing by about half with each additionally favorable level of SES in 1954.
5. *Post-1954 Developments.* None discretely predict women's seeking Treatment.

The corresponding findings for men are as follows:

1. *Demographic Variables.* As in the case of women, the Younger men are about twice more likely to seek Treatment between 1954 and 1974 than the Older men. The chances of the men seeking Treatment increase by about a third with each additional level of favorable Parental SES.
2. *Contexts of Childhood Functioning.* With Demographic Variables and each other controlled, the men's levels of Parental Intrafamily Functioning and Parental Breadwinner Adequacy both predict their seeking Treatment between 1954 and 1974. This is not at all the case among the women.
3. *Pre-Adult Well-Being.* Impairment in childhood is not predictive for the men, although it is for the women.
4. *Baseline Adult Functioning.* Mental Health Impaired men are six and half times more likely than the other men to seek Treatment. This is not the case among the women, for whom simply not being Well was predictive.
5. *Post-1954 Developments.* With all other predictors in the model controlled, the Developments do not predict seeking Treatment.

The path model in the women with each predictor controlled for all other predictors (AIC) makes the following predictions:

1. *Demographic Variables.* Neither predicts help seeking in the women.

2. *Contexts of Childhood Functioning.* No Context had a discrete predictive relationship with seeking Treatment.

3. *Pre-Adult Well-Being.* We find that in the women that level of pre-adult functioning discretely predicts their subsequent help seeking.

4. *Baseline Adult Functioning.* Only the women's level of 1954 SES predicts their seeking Treatment between 1954 and 1974.

5. *Post-1954 Developments.* None discretely predict the women's seeking Treatment.

The corresponding results for men are as follows:

1. *Demographic Variables.* Unlike in the women, in the men both Age level and level of Parental SES predict their seeking Treatment with all other predictors controlled.

2. *Contexts of Childhood Functioning.* Only among the Midtown men does Parental Breadwinner Adequacy discretely predict seeking Treatment. Controlling for all concurrent and antecedent predictors, including the objective level of Parental SES, those men with more favorable levels of Parental Breadwinner Adequacy tended to be more likely to seek Treatment than those with less favorable levels. These are, perhaps, the men whose childhood was not adversely affected by the Great Depression. This is a "sleeper effect."

3. *Pre-Adult Well-Being.* Unlike in the women, no prediction is made in the men.

4. *Baseline Adult Functioning.* Net of all other predictors in the model, the men with Impaired MH54 are more than five and a half times as likely as the other men to seek Treatment between 1954 and 1974.

5. *Post-1954 Developments.* Only the men had a Development which predicts seeking Treatment, their level of increase in Severity of Somatic Disorders from 1954 to 1964.

Summary

We may now evaluate our findings for predictions of seeking Treatment using our findings for predictions of mental health status in 1954 to assess the generalizabiity of the MHIM1 finding that those Midtowners most in need of Treatment did not receive it by 1954. Would this also be true of seeking Treatment by 1974? We found that seeking Treatment was still socially distributed: The most well-off Midtowners as measured by their Own level of SES in 1954 were the most likely to seek Treatment. This was particularly the case among the women, among whom no statistical controls lessened the predictive value of 1954 SES.

Notably the Older women did not seek Treatment in proportion to their needs: Although their levels of MH54 tended to have been less favorable than those of the Younger women, it was the Younger women who were more likely to seek Treatment.

It is also noteworthy that neither 1954 Mental Health Wellness nor Impairment predicted seeking Treatment with controls, including for SES54. Having the social resources to seek Treatment in 1954 and thereafter (as in Kadushin, 1969) was a more powerful predictor than actually having a clinical need for Treatment in 1954 (either by having Impaired Mental Health or less than Well Mental Health).

We further tested the basic propositions of MHIM2 by examining the overall associations and predictions of our mental health model's biopsychosocial predictors. We used the predictions with antecedents and concurrents controlled to make this assessment, comparing predictions of seeking Treatment with predictions of mental health levels in 1954 and 1974.

Among the Midtowners overall, 1954 Mental Health was discretely predicted (AIC) by the interaction between Age level and Gender, Parental SES, Parental Breadwinner Adequacy, Parental Intrafamily Functioning, and Pre-Adult Well-Being. We have now seen that Treatment was discretely predicted by Age level, Parental SES, and Pre-Adult Well-Being; but not by Gender, the interaction of Age level and Gender, Parental Breadwinner Adequacy, or Parental Intrafamily Functioning.

With respect to MH74, we had found the following discrete predictors (AIC): the level of somatic disorders up to 1954; MH54; increases in level of somatic disorders between 1954 and 1964, and between 1964 and 1974; the level of affective episodes between 1954 and 1974; and the level of seeking mental health treatment between 1954 and 1974. The two SES measures, Parental SES and Own level of SES in 1954, canceled each other out when mutually controlled. Either would be discretely predictive of MH74 with the other omitted from the model. We have found, however, that Treatment was not predicted discretely by any of the post-1954 developments, but was predicted discretely by both SES measures (even with each other controlled), as well as Age level and level of Pre-Adult Well-Being.

Thus we conclude that the basic propositions of MHIM2 are substantiated by the findings for Treatment, but to a lesser degree than with MH54 or MH74, since fewer predictions are yielded by the models based on the basic propositions of MHIM2.

We further sought to test these propositions by examining the biopsychosocial predictors of seeking Treatment in different Gender and Age groups. Among the Midtown women, with antecedent and concurrent predictors controlled, 1954 Mental Health was predicted by Age level, Parental SES, Parental Intrafamily Functioning, and Pre-Adult Well-Being. All but Parental Intrafamily Functioning predicted Treatment, as did also Own level of SES in 1954. Thus those Midtown women who had the social resources to seek Treatment did so in proportion to their predictors of 1954 Mental Health. It was the Older women who did not seek Treatment to the extent implied by the predictors of 1954 Mental Health. The basic propositions of MHIM2 are well substantiated by the women's data for Treatment.

It is noteworthy that when the predictive model for Treatment was solved controlling intervening and concurrent predictors, SES54 overrode Parental SES in the Midtown women. Furthermore having a MH54 level less favorable than Well predicted that the women would seek Treatment, but not having an Impaired Mental Health level per se in 1954, which was more characteristic of the Older women than the Younger women or the men. Pre-Adult Well-Being continued to be discretely predictive with these controls.

Among the men, MH54 was predicted by Parental SES, Parental Intrafamily Functioning, and Pre-Adult Well-Being. We now find that their levels of Age, Parental SES, and Parental Intrafamily Functioning discretely predicted seeking Treatment. Parental Breadwinner Adequacy also predicted seeking Treatment among the men, with the degree of favorable recollection of the socioeconomic family environment in childhood predicting the likelihood of seeking Treatment.

Only among the men did a clinically important level of MH54, Impaired, predict seeking Treatment with antecedent and concurrent predictors controlled. We should also have expected to see this among the women. Thus, our conclusion is that the MHIM1 finding—that those who are in most need of Treatment are least likely to receive it—does, to a substantial degree, continue to be applicable in MHIM2 as well. We judge this consistent with the specialized literature summarized in appendix 7.1.

Among the women MH74 was predicted with intervening and concurrent predictors controlled by their levels of MH54, Change in Somatic Disorders from 1954 to 1964, and from 1964 to 1974; and Affective Episodes between 1954 and 1974. With antecedent and concurrent predictors controlled MH74 was predicted among the women by their levels of Age, Parental SES, Parental Intrafamily Functioning, Pre-Adult Well-Being, MH54, Change in Somatic Disorders from 1954 to 1964, and from 1964 to 1974; and Affective Episodes between 1954 and 1974. This strong level of substantiation of the basic propositions of MHIM2 is repeated at a lower level in the data for Treatment. With intervening and concurrent predictors controlled Treatment was predicted among the women only by less favorable than Well levels of MH54 and their levels of Pre-Adult Well-Being, Somatic Disorders up to 1954, and SES54; whereas with antecedent and concurrent predictors controlled Treatment was predicted only by their levels of Age, Parental SES, Pre-Adult Well-Being, and SES54.

Among the men MH74 was discretely predicted with intervening and concurrent predictors controlled by their levels of Somatic Disorders up to 1954, SES54, MH54, and increase in Somatic Disorders between 1964 and 1974. With antecedent and concurrent predictors controlled MH74 was discretely predicted by their levels of Parental SES, Somatic Disorders up to 1954, SES54, MH54, increase in Somatic Disorders between 1964 and 1974, and Treatment. This strong substantiation of the basic propositions of MHIM2 is repeated at an equivalently strong level with the data for Treatment. With intervening and concurrent predictors controlled, Treatment was predicted among the men by Impaired MH54, and by their levels of Age, Parental SES, and Change in Somatic Disorders between 1954 and 1964. Treatment was predicted among the men with antecedent and concurrent predictors controlled by Impaired MH54, and by their levels of Age, Parental SES, Parental Intrafamily Functioning, and Parental Breadwinner Adequacy.

An Evaluation of Mental Health Treatment
by Midtowners Who Sought Help

We have seen that the Midtowners consumed Treatment in a manner which can be predicted from their Sociodemographic Background characteristics, some of their Contexts of Childhood Functioning, their Pre-Adult Well-Being, and their level of 1954 Mental Health (in particular less than Well MH54 in the women and Impaired MH54 in the men). We have also observed that those Midtowner men who sought Treatment between 1954 and 1974 had a less favorable level of MH74 than did those who did not seek treatment, even with the preexisting level of adult mental status, MH54, controlled.

Under Leo Srole's direction, it was part of the Midtown Study tradition to advocate finding out important things about people's lives simply by asking them.[3] Therefore after being asked about whether or not they had sought treatment for mental health problems, Midtowners who had were asked the following:

"All in all, did going to the [(clinic) and (private professional)] make your problem(s)...better, worse, or was there no change?"

Of the 143 Midtowners who reported seeking Treatment, 135 (94 percent) respond to this question. The "Better" response was given by 107 of the 135 Midtowners (79 percent), whereas only 28 Midtowners (21 percent) reported that the treatment resulted in "No Change". Thus eight out of ten of the Midtowners who sought help reported that Treatment helped them.

An additional item was asked, to which all but three of the 135 Midtowners responded:

"Would you say it made your problem(s) a lot, somewhat, or, only a little better?"

We combined these two measures to create an overall measure of the Midtowners' evaluation of how much their treatment helped them. If they said "There was no change," they were assigned a 0 for "Not At All Helped." If they responded "Better," they were assigned a 1 for "A Little," a 2 for "Somewhat," and a 3 for "A Lot." Fully half of the Midtowners who answered both items rated their treatment as "A Lot" helpful (66/132 = 50 percent), while 26 (20 percent) responded "Somewhat," 12 (9 percent) as "A Little" and 28 (21 percent) as "No change (Not At All Helpful)." We abbreviate this measure as HELPED.

Biopsychosocial Predictors and Correlates of Self-Reported Helpfulness of Mental Health Treatment

Two questions of perennial interest to the mental health community are "Who consumes treatment services?" and "Who finds them helpful?" Data from MHIM2 prompts these questions: What might predict "consumer satisfaction" among those who had Treatment[4]? Might the basic propositions of MHIM2 be applicable to this data? Our answers to these questions start with the observed associations of the predicted characteristic, HELPED, and potential predictors. We have chosen to include new potential predictors and socioclinical correlates. Among these is a measure of change in level of affective symptoms from 1954 to 1974.[5]

In the total sample of 132 Midtowners with scores for HELPED, a moderate association shows a trend for Midtowners with higher levels of Affective Episodes between 1954 and 1974 to more favorably rate the helpfulness of Treatment.[6] There was also a moderate trend for Midtowners with more favorable levels of Change in Affective Symptoms to make more favorable ratings of the helpfulness of Treatment.

These associations suggest that Midtowners who are brought to treatment by problems with affect and mood are their clinicians' most satisfied customers.

To further explore the limits of applicability of the basic propositions of MHIM2 we now investigate the Gender-specific predictors and socioclinical correlates of the rated helpfulness of Treatment. Among the women, only three biopsychosocial characteristics are associated with the rated helpfulness of Treatment:

- The higher their level of Body Damage, the less favorable is their rating of Treatment.
- The women who had Treatment and yet had above-average levels of Affective Symptoms in 1974 rate that treatment as less helpful than those who had Treatment and had average- or below-average levels of Affective Symptoms in 1974.
- The more favorable is their Change in Affective Symptoms from 1954 to 1974, the more favorable is their rating of the helpfulness of Treatment.

Whereas among the women only three associations are found out of thirty two potential predictors or socioclinical correlates, among the men ten are statistically significant. Furthermore there is no overlap between these ten and the three in the women.

- The older the men were, the more favorable is their HELPED rating.
- The more favorable the men's level of Parental SES, the more favorable is their HELPED rating.
- The more unfavorable the men's level of Parental Intrafamily Functioning, the more favorably they rate Treatment.
- The more favorable the men's level of Parental Breadwinner Adequacy, the more favorable is their level of HELPED.[7]
- The more extended were the men's Family-Kin Networks in childhood, the more helpful they rate Treatment.
- The less favorable the men's level of Pre-Adult Well-Being, the more helpful they rate Treatment.
- The more favorable the men's level of 1954 SES, the more favorable is their HELPED rating.
- The less favorable the men's level of Affective Episodes, the more favorably they rate HELPED.
- The more favorable their level of Occupation in 1974, the more favorably they rate HELPED.[8]

Among the women there is only one potential predictor of HELPED, Body Damage, and this predictor becomes insignificant in the context of our model of 1974 Mental Health based on the basic propositions of MHIM2. In other words, the model based on the basic propositions of MHIM2 does not predict their HELPED ratings.

Among the men, the model may be predictive. We find with the model controlled for antecedent and concurrent predictors (AC) these predictions:

• The more favorable the men's level of Parental SES, the more favorable is their HELPED rating.
• The less favorable their level of Pre-Adult Well-Being, the more helpful they rate Treatment.
• The more favorable their level of 1954 Mental Health, the more favorable is their HELPED level.
• The more unfavorable their level of Affective Symptoms in 1954, the more favorable is their level of HELPED.

The model in the men controlling for intervening and concurrent predictors (IC) yields the following predictions:

• The more favorable their level of MH54, the more favorable is their HELPED rating.
• The more favorable their level of 1954 SES, the more favorably they rate Treatment.
• The more unfavorable their level of Pre-Adult Well-Being, the more favorable is their rating of HELPED.

We see here that whether it is Parental SES or SES54 being controlled makes a substantial difference in the predictions. Without being controlled for the extent to which it is predicted by Parental SES, SES54 overrides the prediction made above by 1954 Affective Symptom level: the men most likely to rate Treatment as helpful are those who were not below average in the favorableness of their MH54, were above average in their level of SES in 1954, and were below average in their level of Pre-Adult Well-Being.

The predictions made by the model with each predictor controlled for all other predictors (AIC) are as follows:

• The less favorable the men's level of Affective Symptoms in 1954, the more helpful they rate Treatment.
• The more favorable their level of MH54, the more favorable is their HELPED rating.

- The more favorable their level of Pre-Adult Well-Being, the more helpful they rate Treatment.
- The more favorable their level of Parental Breadwinner Adequacy, the more favorably they rate Treatment.

This last prediction is noteworthy, because it suggests that the men's sense of how secure and comfortable their childhood family was predicts the extent to which they can be helped by Treatment: At each level of 1954 SES, those men who had Treatment and had relatively more favorably experienced the socioeconomic status of their childhood family rate the treatment as more helpful than those who had relatively less favorably experienced their childhood SES.

Conclusions

It is known that being physically ill may increase a person's exposure to the mental health system, (e.g., via referral from the treating physician [Regier et al. 1978]), and yet none of our measures of history of somatic disorders (up to 1954, 1954–1964, or 1964–1974), correlates with or predicts seeking Treatment. Having Affective Episodes would also bring the Midtowners into Treatment, one would think, and yet in the total sample this measure also does not correlate with or discretely predict seeking treatment for mental health problems.

We might reasonably conclude from the predictions we have found that Midtowners who have certain Sociodemographic Background characteristics, certain early life experiences, and/or an advantageous level of SES as adults will seek Treatment. Their consumption of Treatment could not be predicted simply from aspects of their 1954 Adult Functioning other than their level of SES in 1954. An additional problem may be that the Midtown women and men sought treatment for mental health problems under different circumstances, with different life historical factors predisposing them to do so.

The women who had some indication (according to MHIM2 data) of a need for Treatment were more likely to obtain it after 1954, although this was not the case in the total panel. The most consistent predictors of the women's seeking Treatment were their levels of Pre-Adult Well-Being and Own SES in 1954. There was also one indication that the women with less favorable than Well levels of MH54 were more likely to seek Treatment than the women with Well MH54.

The men produced quite different data for Treatment: Regardless of controls, an Impaired level of MH54 predicted a higher chance of seeking Treatment than more favorable levels of MH54. Younger men were more likely to seek Treatment than Older men, regardless of controls; but there were some indications of this Age association among the women as well. Men with more favorable levels of Parental SES showed a trend towards a higher chance of seeking Treatment than men with less favorable levels; but here too there were some indications of this among the women. Finally among the men, but not among the women, there were some indications that an unfavorable level of change in somatic disorders between 1954 and 1964 predicted seeking Treatment.

The models implied by the basic propositions of MHIM2 applied at least as well to the Treatment data for the men as to their data for MH54 and MH74, given the spectrum of biopsychosocial predictions we found. But by the same criteria, among the women the applicability to the Treatment data was at a lesser level than among the men.

The findings for the models as applied to predicting whether Midtowners who sought Treatment found it helpful unequivocally indicate that the ratings of Midtown men were substantially explained by the models, although at a lesser level than was the case with their levels of MH54 and MH74, judging from the number of associations and predictions obtained in our analyses. No understanding of the women's ratings is contributed by these models.

Did the MHIM1 finding that those Midtowners most need of Treatment were the least likely to obtain it generalize to MHIM2? We have found the following trends towards its generalizability:

- Midtowners with more favorable levels of SES54 are more likely to seek Treatment than those with less favorable levels, yet those with less favorable levels of SES54 had a greater need for Treatment as shown by their less favorable levels of MH74. This is particularly the case for the Midtown women, who not only show the association found among the men but have their seeking Treatment predicted by SES54 regardless of statistical controls.

- Younger Midtowners are more likely to seek Treatment than Older Midtowners, but the need for Treatment of the Older Midtowners is at least as great as the need of the Younger Midtowners. Among men in particular, the prediction is made by Age level regardless of statistical controls; but there is an association among women that survives one set of statistical controls (AC).

- Midtowners from more favorable Parental SES levels are more likely to seek Treatment than those from less favorable Parental SES levels, yet the latter had a greater need for Treatment as indicated by trends for MH54 and MH74. Again this prediction is made among the men in particular regardless of statistical controls; but there is an association among women that survives one set of statistical controls (AC).

- Midtown women whose MH54 level is Impaired are not more likely than those whose MH54 levels are more favorable to seek Treatment. But there were some indications that women whose MH54 level is less favorable than Well are more likely to seek Treatment than those whose MH54 level is Well.

But we also found trends suggesting the limits of the generalizability of the MHIM1 finding to MHIM2 given the expansion of the mental health treatment system, including service provision and funding, between 1954 and 1974:

- Midtowners with less favorable levels of Pre-Adult Well-Being may be considered to have a greater need for Treatment than those with more favorable levels. Among Midtowners overall, those whose levels of Pre-Adult Well-Being are less favorable are more likely to seek Treatment than those whose levels are more favorable. Among Midtowners overall and particularly among the women, this prediction is obtained regardless of statistical controls; but the overall association is also shown by the men.
- Midtowner men with Impaired MH54 are more likely to seek Treatment than the men with more favorable levels of MH54, regardless of statistical controls. From a clinical point of view they are in the most need of Treatment. No such trend is seen among the women.
- Midtowner women whose MH54 level is less favorable than Well are more likely to seek Treatment than those whose MH54 level is Well. This may be seen as a relatively weak indication that the women who need Treatment seek it.

We are more impressed by the trends suggesting that the MHIM1 finding generalizes to MHIM2. In particular these trends suggest that although some men with Impaired MH54 seek Treatment, the odds are they also had more favorable SES characteristics. Whether the impact of the managed care revolution on the availability of mental health treatment to those most in need will be positive or negative is an imperative subject for future public mental health research.

Notes

1. See Appendix 7.1 for further discussion of these extremely important studies.
2. We realize that there is some danger in considering the three other Post-1954 Developments to be true predictors of mental health treatment—they might just as accurately be regarded as reciprocal to seeking Treatment. We decided to include the Developments as predictors because clinical experience as well as epidemiological research has well established that people often seek mental health

treatment when they experience emotional instability, and/or when their physical health status deteriorates. Research supports this interpretation to such an extent that we present a specialized bibliography in appendix 7.1. Furthermore, by including the three other Developments as predictors we can control antecedent predictors for their paths to these Developments. Thus it is all the more surprising that these predictors do not predict help seeking in the panel.

3. For example, the Midtown Study, in 1954, was the first to simply ask community residents about their overall health status: "About your health now, would you say it is: excellent, good, fair, or poor?" Responses to this item predict whether the Midtowner would be found deceased by 1974 (Singer et al. 1976) even when levels of Age, Gender, Mental Health in 1954, Marital Status in 1954, SES in 1954, and a summary measure of eight somatic disorders (including the Midtowners' reports of diabetes, high blood pressure, heart condition, smoking, obesity, ulcers, colitis, and alcohol drinking) are controlled.

4. This is, for example, a major concern of health agencies ranging from the Alliance for the Mentally Ill to the Joint Commission for the Accreditation of Healthcare Organizations.

5. This measure compares the observed level of affective symptoms in 1974 with the expected level based on the 1954 level. See the Statistical Appendices for further details. The 1974 level of affective symptoms is measured from the same items as the 1954 level, as replicated in the MHIM2 interview.

6. This may be viewed as a socioclinical correlate of Treatment rather than a predictor, as well as the kindred variables which immediately follow.

7. Specifically a group of ten Midtowners who scored in the least favorable level of Parental Breadwinner Adequacy and had mental health treatment reported a lower level of benefit than the other Midtowners who had mental health treatment.

8. The 1974 measure of level of Occupation was developed by Leo Srole and Lirio Covey from items in the 1974 interview. This and measures of 1974 levels of Income and Education replicated the 1954 measures. A measure of 1974 level of Social Network Density was developed in parallel to the 1954 level, from MHIM2 interview items, by Leo Srole and Jackson Kytle. Note that the terms "density" and "extensivity" are synonymous with respect to our measure of Social Network.

Appendix 7.1

References with Comments

Since MHIM1, the research literature regarding seeking health care and medical treatment has burgeoned. In this Appendix we shall list some studies which we have reviewed, sometimes specifying which findings of these studies are especially notable for MHIM2.

Anderson, Ronald M. "Revisiting the behavioral model and access to medical care: does it matter?" *Journal of Health and Social Behavior* 36 (March 1995): 1–10.

Broman, Clifford L., William S. Hoffman, and V. Lee Hamilton. "Impact of mental health services use on subsequent mental health of autoworkers." *Journal of Health and Social Behavior* 35 (March 1994): 80–94.

We noted in particular this study's finding that autoworkers who consumed Treatment showed higher levels of psychological problems afterwards than those who did not seek Treatment. There were indications that this unfavorable effect was especially seen among African American, older, poorly educated, and/or unemployed autoworkers.

Bush, Patricia J. and Marian Osterweis. "Pathways to medicine use." *Journal of Health and Social Behavior* 19 (June 1978): 179–89.

Fox, John W. "Sex, marital status, and age as social selection factors in recent psychiatric treatment." *Journal of Health and Social Behavior* 25 (December 1984): 394–405.

Janz, Nancy and Marshall Becker. "The health belief model: a decade later." *Health Education Quarterly*, 11 (Spring 1984): 1–47.

The Health Belief Model has been an extremely influential paradigm, which applies social psychological concepts to the entire domain of health-related behavior, including seeking treatment and compliance with healthcare regimens. It has been so extensively researched that alternative models have been proposed which perhaps better account for the relationships among the components of the model.

Kadushin, Charles. 1969. *Why People Go to Psychiatrists.* New York: Atherton.

———. "The friends and supporters of psychotherapy: on social circles in urban life." *American Sociological Review* 31 (December 1966): 786–802.

These two contributions by one of the graduate school professors of the present junior author broke new ground in empirically establishing that the reasons for Manhattan residents seeking Treatment had nothing to do with any potential objective mental health needs, but rather reflected their location in Manhattan society, e.g., their social resources.

Miller, William R. "Motivation for treatment: a review with special emphasis on alcoholism." *Psychological Bulletin* 98 (July 1985): 84–108.

This review article was an important step towards the development of the "motivational interviewing" clinical technique, presented in the following monograph:

Miller, William R. 1991. *Motivational Interviewing: Preparing People to Change Addictive Behavior.* New York: Guilford Press

Portes, Alejandro, David Kyle, and William W. Eaton. "Mental illness and help-seeking behavior among Mariel Cuban and Haitian refugees in South Florida." *Journal of Health and Social Behavior* 33 (December 1992): 283–98.

Regier, Darrel A., Irving Goldberg and Carl A. Taube. "The De Facto U.S. Mental Health Services System: A Public Health Perspective." *Archives of General Psychiatry* 35 (June 1978): 685–93.

Shapiro, Sam, Elizabeth A. Skinner, Larry G. Kessler, Michael Von Korff, Pearl S. German, Gary L. Tischler, Philip J. Leaf, Lee Benham, Linda Cottler, and Darrel A. Regier. "Utilization of health and mental health services." *Archives of General Psychiatry* 41 (October 1984): 971–78.

This article presents data from the first of the large sample modern mental health surveys, the Epidemiological Catchment Area study of the early 1980s. Although the senior author had reservations about the methods used in this study, a data collection of this magnitude merits the full attention of the interested reader.

Veroff, Joseph, Elizabeth Douvan and Richard A. Kulka. 1981. *The Inner American: A Self-Portrayal from 1957 to 1976*. New York: Basic Books.

This extremely important, best-selling monograph set the stage for these authors' next monograph, examining the seeking of mental health treatment. Among their many findings, the following struck us as especially noteworthy: (1) Subjective well-being levels reported by the 1976 respondents did not substantially differ from those reported by the 1954 respondents. (2) Younger 1976 respondents were the most likely to identify their childhoods as the time in their lives they were most unhappy. (3) Women rate their well-being more unfavorably than do men. (4) Better educated respondents were more likely to seek Treatment than the less educated, yet also were more likely to rate their well-being more favorably than the less educated. (5) The stage of the adult life cycle in which both the 1957 and 1976 respondents were in forms a pervasive and influential context for their self-ratings of well-being. (6) Trends from these surveys did not indicate Generational differences ("cohort effects"). (7) Age level, but not Generation, predicts ratings of well-being, although sometimes in a Gender-specific manner.

MHIM2 also finds that the (same) respondents, our Midtowners, reported levels of mental health characteristics in 1974 no different, on the average, than those from those characteristics in 1954. Both of our socioeconomic measures, Parental level and Own level in 1954, are pervasively associated and predictive of mental health characteristics. There is a weak trend for the women to report less favorable levels of mental health characteristics than do the men in 1954, but this is not found in 1974. Further analysis shows that it is the Older women who produce this trend. Impaired childhood well-being is quite consequential for adult mental health characteristics in MHIM2 data. Finally, and in a most remarkably different manner than in the Veroff et al. study, MHIM2 data for mental health shows a marked Generational effect, which this monograph has fully described. Further statistical details and data are available in the Statistical Appendices.

Veroff, Joseph, Richard A. Kulka and Elizabeth Douvan. 1981. *Mental Health in America: Patterns of Help Seeking from 1957 to 1976*. New York: Basic Books.

This best-selling monograph was an epochal achievement. We particularly noted the following findings: (1) Although the spectrum of problems which prompted 1976 respondents to seek Treatment was about the same as those of 1957 respondents, the prominence of marriage problems diminished from 1957 to 1976. This change is especially noted among respondents who were divorced or separated in 1957 or 1976. (2) On the basis of the types of problems which bring their 1957 and 1976 respondents into Treatment, Veroff et al. differentiate among four patterns of seeking Treatment: (a) both a personal problem and a crisis, (b) only a personal problem, (c) only a crisis, and (d) for neither a personal problem nor a crisis. Somatic disorders account for a plurality of crises driving respondents to seek Treatment, and for a substantial fraction of personal problems.

Additional References

Fischer, Anita K., Janos Marton, Ernest J. Millman, and Leo Srole. 1979. "Long-range influences on adult mental health: The Midtown Manhattan Longitudinal Study, 1954–1974," in *Research in Community and Mental Health, vol. 1*, edited by Roberta G. Simmons, 305–33. Greenwich, CT: JAI Press.

Singer, Eleanor, Robin Garfinkel, Steven M. Cohen, and Leo Srole. "Mortality and Mental Health: The Midtown Manhattan Restudy." *Social Science and Medicine* 10 (November 1976): 517–25.

Srole, Leo, Thomas S. Langner, Stanley T. Michael, Price Kirkpatrick, Marvin K. Opler, and Thomas A. C. Rennie. 1975. *Mental Health in the Metropolis: The Midtown Manhattan Study*. Enlarged and revised edition, edited by Leo Srole and Anita K. Fischer. New York: Harper and Row Torchbooks.

8

Other Aspects of Change in Adult Health
from 1954 to 1974

We have tested the basic propositions of MHIM2 with the longitudinal data for global mental health and use of mental health treatment, and have found that these propositions are well substantiated. In this chapter, we continue our exploration of the basic propositions with the data for other aspects of adult health, to describe the extent to which these other aspects are predicted by the models of mental health implied by the basic propositions.

Our objectives in this chapter are as follows:

1. To describe the associations among 1954 levels of adult functioning measures in the total sample, and in each Gender separately.

2. To describe the associations among 1974 levels of adult functioning measures in the total sample, and in each Gender separately.

3. To show the extent to which change in the Midtowners' socioeconomic status from childhood to their own level in 1954 predicts changes in adult functioning between 1954 and 1974.

4. To describe our path analysis of level of Affective Symptoms, beginning with 1954 levels, and the 1974 levels.

5. To describe the findings our path analyses of the three remaining Post-1954 Developments. These are:
   • Level of Increase in the Severity of Somatic Disorders between 1954 and 1964.
   • Level of Increase in the Severity of Somatic Disorders between 1964 and 1974.
   • Level of Affective Episodes.

6. To describe all of these path analyses first for the total sample and then for each Gender separately.

7. To describe our path analysis of each new aspect of Generation-separated levels of adult health, first for the total sample and then for each Gender separately.

Associations among Measures of 1954 Adult Functioning

In the data for the total panel of Midtowners, we find associations between their levels of Mental Health and their 1954 levels of Affective Symptoms, Social Network Density, Excess Intake, and Socioeconomic Status. Among the Midtown women and men separately, we find the same pattern of associations.[1]

Associations among Measures of 1974 Adult Functioning

When we examine the associations among three socioeconomic status measures—Income, Occupation, and Education—and 1974 levels of Affective Symptoms, Social Network Extensivity, Excess Intake, and Global Mental Health, we find the following patterns: (1) There was a tendency for higher levels of Occupation, Income, Education, and Social Network Extensivity to be associated. These variables are indicative of socioeconomic functioning. (2) There is a tendency for less favorable levels of Mental Health (MH) to be associated with less favorable levels of Excessive Intakes and Affective Symptoms. These variables are indicative of adult mental health functioning. We find overall an association indicating that as levels of socioeconomic functioning become more favorable, levels of adult mental health functioning become more favorable.

When we review the associations among the women alone, we find, with two exceptions, the same pattern of associations as in the total sample. Those exceptions involve no association between levels of MH74 and social network extensivity; and none between 1974 levels of Affective Disorders and Occupation. Among the men, 1974 levels of Affective Symptoms and Occupation are associated, as are those between their levels of MH74 and social network extensivity. However, only among the women is there an association between their 1974 level of Excess Intake and MH74.

Social Mobility and Later Changes in Adult Functioning

In chapter 4 we discussed how we measure social mobility from the level of Parental Socioeconomic Status (SES) to the level of Own SES in 1954 by multiplying one SES measure by the other, and then controlling for each SES measure to estimate the prediction of a characteristic of our subjects by their social mobility. This measure is, of course, concurrent with the 1954 Adult Functioning measures, but may be a predictor of post-1954 Adult Functioning. Here we review the extent to which social mobility might predict those measures.

We begin by reviewing the interaction associations between the level of social mobility and measures of post-1954 Adult Functioning, finding that social mobility predicts only the 1974 level of Affective Symptoms and 1974 level of Income.[2] Accordingly, we add to the basic model of mental health derived from the basic propositions of MHIM2, the interaction association when we analyze 1974 level of Affective Symptoms.

When we closely examine the nature of the interaction association with 1974 level of Affective Symptoms we find that Midtowners who fall in the High-High level of Parental SES who did not achieve an Own SES level in 1954 of High-High have less favorable levels than those who did achieve the High-High level in 1954.

Among the Midtown women, social mobility predicts their 1974 level of Affective Symptoms, Social Network Density, Income, and Occupation. Predictions of the women's Social Network Density level in 1974 and 1974 Occupational level are not seen in the total sample. Among the men, social mobility predicts their 1974 levels of Income and Occupation. Men do not show the prediction by social mobility of 1974 Affective Symptom level seen in the total sample, or the prediction of Social Network Density level in 1974 found in the women.

Predictions of Adult Health by Sociodemographic Background, Contexts of Childhood Functioning, Pre-Adult Well-Being, and Severity of Somatic Disorders up to 1954

We extend our exploration of the basic propositions of MHIM2 by seeing the extent to which the life-span models of mental health derived from them apply to each aspect of Adult Health, starting with its 1954 level, proceeding to its 1974 level, and finally to the change in its level from 1954 to 1974.

Level of Affective Symptoms

1954 Level of Affective Symptoms. Most of the model predictors are associated, with the exceptions of Gender, Age level, and level of extensivity of Family-Kin Networks. Among the Midtown women, only their levels of Body Damage and Family-Kin Network are not associated. In contrast to the women, only the men's levels of Parental level of SES and Pre-Adult Well-Being are associated.

In the total panel of Midtowners, 1954 level of Affective Symptoms is consistently predicted by their levels of Parental SES and Pre-Adult Well-Being (AC, IC, and AIC). There are some indications, depending on which model is used (AC or IC), that other biopsychosocial predictors including Parental Intrafamily Functioning (AC), Parental Bread-winner Adequacy (IC), and level of Severity of Somatic Disorders up to 1954 (IC) may be predictive. About 5 percent of 1954 level of Affective Symptoms is predicted by the model of mental health (MH) based on the basic propositions of MHIM2, much less than the 21 percent of 1954 MH predicted by the model. Among the women, Age level and level of Pre-Adult Well-Being are consistently predictive (AC, IC, and AIC). There are some indications, as in the total panel, that Parental Intrafamily Functioning (AC), Parental Breadwinner Adequacy (AC and IC), and level of Severity of Somatic Disorders up to 1954 (IC) may be predictive. About 6 percent of 1954 Affective Symptom levels in the women is predicted by the model, much less than the 24 percent of MH54 so predicted. Among the men, only Parental level of SES is consistently predictive (AC, IC, and AIC). As in the total panel and the women, there is an indication that Pre-Adult Well-Being may be predictive (IC). The model does not predict the 1954 Affective Symptom levels in the men, whereas it predicts 15 percent of their MH54 levels.

1974 Level of Affective Symptoms. When we review the associations of Affective Symptom level in 1974 and its potential biopsychosocial predictors, associations are observed in the total sample between Affective Symptom level in 1974 and Age level, Parental level of SES, Pre-Adult Well-Being, all of the 1954 Adult Functioning measures except level of Excess Intakes, and the level of increase in Severity of Somatic Disorders between 1964 and 1974. In the women, Affective Symptom level in 1974 is associated with Age level, Parental level of SES, Pre-Adult Well-Being, all of the 1954 Adult Functioning measures except level of Excess Intakes, the level of increase in Severity of Somatic Disorders between 1964 and 1974, and Mental Health Treatment. But in the men, in contrast, Affective Symptom level in 1974 is associated only with Affective Symptom level in 1954, level of Severity of Somatic Disorders up to 1954, and the level of increase in Severity of Somatic Disorders between 1964 and 1974.

In the total panel of Midtowners, levels of Pre-Adult Well-Being, Severity of Somatic Disorders up to 1954, 1954 Affective Symptoms, and Social Mobility consistently predict their 1974 levels of Affective Symptoms.[3] In addition, depending upon the model, there are indications that levels of Age (AC), Parental SES (AC), SES54 (IC), change in Severity of Somatic Disorders from 1964 to 1974 (AC and IC), and Treatment (AC and AIC) may predict 1974 levels of Affective Symptoms. About 21 percent of levels in 1974 Affective Symptoms is predicted by the model of mental health based on the basic propositions of MHIM2, somewhat less than the 29 percent of levels of MH74 explained by the model.

Among the Midtown women, levels of Pre-Adult Well-Being, 1954 Affective Symptoms, and Social Mobility consistently predict their 1974 level of Affective Symptoms. In addition, depending upon which approach is used, the women's levels of Age (AC), Parental SES (AC), Severity of Somatic Disorders up to 1954 (AC and AIC), increase in Severity of Somatic Disorders between 1964 and 1974 (IC), and Treatment (AC and AIC) predict 1974 levels of Affective Symptoms. The model of mental health based upon the basic propositions of MHIM2 predicts about 20 percent of the women's levels of 1974 Affective Symptoms, much less than the 32 percent of the women's levels of MH74 predicted by the model.

Largely consistent with the findings in the women, the men's levels of 1974 Affective Symptoms are consistently predicted by their 1954 level of Affective Symptoms, Severity of Somatic Disorders up to 1954, and Social Mobility. With different models there are some indications that the men's levels of Pre-Adult Well-Being (AC), and change in Severity of Somatic Disorders from 1964 to 1974 (IC) predict their 1974 Affective Symptom level. About the same percentage of the men's 1974 levels of Affective Symptoms, 23 percent, is predicted by the model as in the women (20 percent). For the men only, the level of prediction of 1974 Affective Symptoms is about the same as for MH74 (24 percent).

Increase in Severity of Somatic Disorders from 1954 to 1964

When we look at the associations between the increase in the level of Severity of Somatic Disorders from 1954 to 1964 and potential biopsychosocial predictors in the total panel of Midtowners, we see trends for levels of Age, Body Damage, and Severity of Somatic Disorders up to 1954.

In the total panel, SES54 consistently predicts the increase in level of Severity from 1954 to 1964 although without controls SES54 was not associated with that measure of change.[4] There are indications that increase in Severity may be predicted by levels of Age (AC and IC), Body Damage (AC and AIC), and Severity up to 1954 (IC). The model of mental health derived from the basic propositions of MHIM2 predicts about 5 percent of the levels of increase in level of Severity. Among the women, the model does not at all predict increase in level of Severity. Among the men, levels of SES54 and Severity of Somatic Disorder up to 1954 consistently predict increase in Severity. The trends are for the less socioeconomically advantaged Midtown men to have greater levels of increase in Severity and for Midtown men who had more unfavorable levels of Severity up to 1954 to have greater increases in Severity between 1954 and 1964. There are some indications that levels of Family-Kin Network Extensivity (AC and AIC) may predict increase in Severity between 1954 and 1964.

Increase in Severity of Somatic Disorders from 1964 to 1974

In the total panel of Midtowners, increase in Severity from 1964 to 1974 is associated with levels of Age, Gender, Severity of Somatic Disorders up to 1954, MH54, SES54, and increase in Severity from 1954 to 1964. Among the Midtown women, increase from 1964 to 1974 is associated with levels of Age, Body Damage, Parental Intrafamily Functioning, Family-Kin Network extensivity, Severity up to 1954, MH54, 1954 Affective Symptoms, and increase in Severity from 1954 to 1964. But among the men, only levels of Age and SES54 are associated with increase in Severity from 1964 to 1974.

In the total panel of Midtowners, increase in Severity of Somatic Disorders between 1964 and 1974 is consistently predicted by levels of Age (the Older tend to have greater increases than the Younger), SES54 (the more disadvantaged tend to have greater increases than the more advantages), and increase between 1954 and 1964 (the Midtowners who had greater increases between 1954 and 1964 had greater increases between 1964 and 1974 as well). There are also some indications, depending upon the model used, that the level of Severity up to 1954 (IC) and MH54 (IC) may predict increase between 1964 and 1974, in the expected direction (the more unfavorable the level up to 1954, the greater the increase in Severity). About 6 percent of levels of increase in Severity are predicted by the model of mental health derived from the basic propositions of MHIM2.

Among the Midtown women, only the level of increase in Severity of Somatic Disorders between 1954 and 1964 consistently predicts the level of increase between 1964 and 1974. In addition there are trends for levels of Age (AC), Parental Intrafamily Functioning (AC), and MH54 (IC) to sometimes predict level of change between 1964 and 1974. These life-span models derived from the basic propositions of MHIM2 predict about 6 percent of the levels of increase among the women in Severity between 1954 and 1964.

The results for the Midtown men are quite different: both levels of Age and SES54 consistently predict level of increase in Severity between 1964 and 1974, and there are no trends for other biopsychosocial characteristics of the men to predict increase. Although the findings are different than for the women, the predictive performance of the model is about the same, 6 percent.

Level of Affective Episodes

In the total panel of Midtowners, increasingly unfavorable levels of Affective Episodes between 1954 and 1974 are associated with increasingly unfavorable levels of Body Damage, Parental Intrafamily Functioning, Pre-Adult Well-Being, MH54, 1954 Affective Symptoms, and Excess Intakes in 1954. Finally, Younger Midtowners tend to have more Affective Episodes than did Older Midtowners. All but two of these associations are found among the Midtown women (the exceptions being Body Damage and 1954 Affective Symptoms). In contrast, levels of Affective Episodes among the Midtown men are associated only with Body Damage and Parental Intrafamily Functioning.

The life-span model derived from the basic propositions of MHIM2 predicts 5 percent of the levels of Affective Episodes, about the same of prediction as the 9 percent of Change in MH. Affective Episodes are predicted by levels of Age, Body Damage, Parental Intrafamily Functioning, and Pre-Adult Well-Being in both the AC and IC models; but when the control for the Age-and-Sex interaction prediction is added (AIC), then only Body Damage level predicts Episodes: Midtowners who have increasingly unfavorable levels of Body Damage tend to have more Episodes than the Midtowners with no Body Damage.

Among the women, Episodes are consistently predicted by Age level. Notably, their levels of Pre-Adult Well-Being predict Episodes in both the AC and IC models. About 8 percent of the level of Episodes is predicted by the life-span model derived from the basic propositions of MHIM2 among the women.

Among the men, the life-span model does not predict levels of Episodes. Nonetheless consistent predictions are found for levels of Age and SES54: Younger men tend to have more Episodes than Older men. Men whose SES54 is increasingly favorable have increasingly favorable levels of Episodes.

Generational Differences in Adult Level of Functioning

We continue our analysis by looking at comparisons of the levels of Generation-separated measures of adult health and other aspects of functioning characterizing the Later and Earlier Generations[5] in the total sample.

- The Earlier Generation has less favorable levels than does the Later Generation of the Generation-separated measures of Affective Symptoms, Mental Health, and Income.
- The Earlier Generation has more favorable levels of the Generation-separated level of Occupation than does the Later Generation. We shall see that this is primarily due to a Generational difference in the women, and not in the men.
- Only the Generation-separated measure of Social Network Density does not feature a Generational difference.

A comparison in the women of the Generation-separated measures of adult functioning between the Later and Earlier Generations yields about the same results as in the total sample. But comparison in the men of Generation-separated measures of adult functioning between the Later and Earlier Generations tells a different story. Unlike in the women, the men do not manifest a Generational difference in their level of Affective Symptoms, Mental Health, or Occupational level. Otherwise their results are the same as for both the women and the total sample.

Generational Differences in Affective Symptoms

In the total panel of Midtowners, when each predictor is controlled for its associations with antecedent and concurrent predictors (AC), the life-span model derived from the basic propositions of MHIM2 makes the following predictions: (1) the Earlier Generation (aged 40–59 years in 1954) has a higher average level of Affective Symptoms than does the Later Generation (aged 40–59 in 1974); (2) the more favorable the Midtowners' level of Parental SES, the more favorable their level of Affective Symptoms at age 40–59; (3) the more favorable the Midtowners' level of Pre-Adult Well-Being, the more favorable their level of Affective Symptoms at age 40–59; (4) the more favorable the Midtowners' level of Severity of Somatic Disorders up to 1954, the more favorable their level of Affective Symptoms at age 40–59.

The model of Generation-separated level of Affective Symptoms with intervening and concurrent predictors controlled (IC) makes the following predictions: (1) the higher the Midtowners' Generation-separated level of Severity of Somatic Disorders, the higher their Generation-separated level of Affective Symptoms; (2) the more favorable the Midtowners' level of Pre-Adult Well-Being, the more favorable their Generation-separated level of Affective Symptoms; (3) the Age-by-Sex interaction predicts that the older the women, the more unfavorable is their Generation-separated level of Affective Symptoms. It is valid to interpret this as indicating that the women's level of Affective Symptoms is, on the average, less favorable in the Earlier Generation than in the Later Generation, consistent with the finding for the Impaired level of Generation-separated MH in women presented in the preceding chapter. The model of Generation-separated level of Affective Symptoms with antecedent, intervening and concurrent predictors controlled (AIC) finds that the Midtowners' level of Affective Symptoms is predicted by their levels of Pre-Adult Well-Being, Severity of Somatic Disorders up to 1954, and the Age-by-Sex interaction, in the expected directions. About 7 percent of levels of Generation-separated Affective Symptoms is explained by the basic model of mental health derived from the basic propositions of MHIM2, moderately less than the 17 percent of levels of Generation-separated MH predicted by that model.

The model of Generation-separated level of Affective Symptoms in the women makes three predictions when each predictor is controlled for its associations with antecedent and concurrent predictors (AC): (1) the average Generation-separated level of Affective Symptoms of the Earlier Generation of the women is less favorable than that of the Later Generation of the women; (2) the more favorable the women's level of Parental SES, the more favorable their Generation-separated level of Affective Symptoms; (3) the more favorable the women's level of Pre-Adult Well-Being, the more favorable their Generation-separated level of Affective Symptoms.

Solving the model with intervening and concurrent predictors controlled (IC) yields two predictions: (1) the more favorable their level of Pre-Adult Well-Being, the more favorable their level of Affective Symptoms; (2) the Earlier women have a less favorable level of Affective Symptoms than do the Later women. The model with antecedent, intervening, and concurrent predictors controlled (AIC) shows that Affective Symptoms are predicted by levels of Age and Pre-Adult Well-Being in the expected direction. The predictive power of the life-span model derived from the basic propositions of MHIM2 is about the same for Generation-separated levels of Affective Symptoms as for MH, about nine percent and eleven percent respectively.

The model of Generation-separated level of Affective Symptoms in the men makes one prediction when each predictor is controlled for its associations with antecedent and concurrent predictors (AC): the more favorable the men's level of Pre-Adult Well-Being, the more favorable is their Generation-separated level of Affective Symptoms. The model with intervening and concurrent predictors controlled (IC) makes the same prediction. The model with antecedent, intervening, and concurrent predictors controlled (AIC) makes this prediction as well. Only in the women is Age level also consistently predictive, an alternative demonstration of the Generation-by-Gender interaction seen in the total panel. The model of mental health derived from the basic propositions of MHIM2 does not predict Generation-separated Affective Symptoms among the men, although it predicts nine percent of levels of MH.

In chapter 7 we presented Generation- and Gender-specific analyses of the Generation-separated measure of Mental Health, in an exploration of the Generation- and Gender-specific difference in the prediction of Mental Health. It is of value, in testing the extent to which the life-span model derived from the basic propositions of MHIM2 is generalizable to other health outcomes, to see how the Generation-separated measure of Affective Symptoms is predicted by that model in each Gender.

The model of Generation-separated level of Affective Symptoms in Earlier women makes two predictions with each predictor controlled for its associations with antecedent and concurrent predictors (AC): (1) The more favorable the Earlier Generation of women's level of Parental Breadwinner Adequacy in childhood, the more favorable their Generation-separated level of Affective Symptoms. (2) The more favorable the Earlier Generation of women's level of Pre-Adult Well-Being, the more favorable their Generation-separated level of Affective Symptoms. The model in Earlier women with intervening and concurrent predictors controlled (IC) makes the same two predictions, while the model with antecedent, intervening, and concurrent predictors controlled (AIC) finds that only their level of Pre-Adult Well-Being consistently predicts their level of Generation-separated Affective

Symptoms. About 7 percent of levels of Generation-separated Affective Symptoms are predicted by the model of mental health derived from the basic model of MHIM2, about the same as the 11 percent of Generation-separated MH predicted among the women overall. But that model does not predict levels of Generation-separated Affective Symptoms in Earlier men.

The model of Generation-separated level of Affective Symptoms in Later women makes two predictions when each predictor is controlled for its associations with antecedent and concurrent predictors (AC): (1) the more favorable the Later Generation of women's level of Pre-Adult Well-Being, the more favorable their Generation-separated level of Affective Symptoms; (2) the more unfavorable the Later Generation of women's Generation-separated level of Severity of Somatic Disorders, the more unfavorable their Generation-separated level of Affective Symptoms. The model of Generation-separated level of Affective Symptoms in Later women with intervening and concurrent predictors controlled (IC) makes these two predictions as well. The model of Generation-separated level of Affective Symptoms in Later women with antecedent, intervening, and concurrent predictors controlled (AIC) yields only the same prediction as made in the Earlier women, namely that by their level of Pre-Adult Well-Being.

The findings that are distinct for the Generations of women are that (1) among the Earlier women only, the less favorable their level of Parental Breadwinner Adequacy, the less favorable their level of Affective Symptoms (in 1954); and (2) among the Later women only, the less favorable their level of Severity of Somatic Disorders up to 1974, the less favorable their level of Affective Symptoms (in 1974).

The model does not predict levels of Generation-separated Affective Symptoms in the Later Generation of men. However, there is a suggestive trend for the prediction that the more favorable the Later Generation of men's level of Pre-Adult Well-Being, the more favorable their Generation-separated level of Affective Symptoms.

We conclude that level of Pre-Adult Well-Being is the single discrete predictor of levels of the Generation-separated measure of Affective Symptoms for all Midtowners except the Earlier men.

Generational Differences in Level of Severity of Somatic Disorders

The model of Generation-separated level of Severity of Somatic Disorders makes the following predictions when each predictor's associations with antecedent and concurrent predictors is controlled (AC): (1) the women have a higher Generation-separated level of Severity of Somatic Disorders than do the men; (2) the Later Generation of Midtowners has a higher Generation-separated level of Severity than does the Earlier Generation[6]; (3) the more unfavorable the Midtowners' level of Body Damage, the higher their Generation-separated level of Severity of Somatic Disorders; (4) the more unfavorable the Midtowners' level of Pre-Adult Well-Being, the more unfavorable their Generation-separated level of Severity. The model of Generation-separated level of Severity of Somatic Disorders with intervening and concurrent predictors controlled (IC) makes three predictions: (1) The more favorable the Midtowners' level of Pre-Adult Well-Being, the more favorable their Generation-separated level of Severity. (2) The more unfavorable their level of Body Damage in childhood, the less favorable their Generation-separated level of Severity. (3) The Later Generation has a less favorable Generation-separated average level of Severity than does the Earlier Generation. The model of Generation-separated level of Severity of Somatic Disorders with antecedent, intervening, and concurrent predictors controlled (AIC) finds the three same predictions.

It is striking that although there is no overall Gender difference in Generation-separated level of Severity of Somatic Disorders, when Age is controlled in the AC model the two Genders show different levels: specifically, the women tend to have higher levels than the men when Age level is controlled. The life-span model derived from the basic propositions of MHIM2 predicts 8 percent of the levels of Generation-separated Severity, somewhat less than the 17 percent predicted of levels of Generation-separated MH.

The model of Generation-separated level of Severity of Somatic Disorders in the women with the associations of each predictor with antecedent and concurrent predictors controlled (AC) makes the following predictions: (1) The Later Generation of the women has a more unfavorable average Generation-separated level of Severity than does the Earlier Generation. (2) The more unfavorable the women's level of Body Damage in childhood, the more unfavorable their Generation-separated level of Severity. (3) The more unfavorable the women's level of Parental Intrafamily Functioning in childhood, the more unfavorable their Generation-separated level of Severity. (4) The more unfavorable the women's level of Parental Breadwinner Adequacy, the more unfavorable their Generation-separated level of Severity. The model with intervening and concurrent predictors controlled (IC) makes four predictions: (1) the more favorable the women's level of Pre-Adult Well-Being, the more favorable their Generation-separated level of Severity; (2) the more favorable the women's level of Body Damage in Childhood, the more favorable their Generation-separated level of Severity; (3) the more favorable the women's level of Parental Intrafamily Functioning, the more favorable their Generation-separated level of Severity; (4) the Later Generation of women has a less favorable average Generation-separated level of Severity than does the Earlier Generation. The model with antecedent, intervening, and concurrent predictors controlled (AIC) shows that consistent predictions are made by their levels of Generation, Body Damage, and Parental Intrafamily Functioning. The power of the life-span model derived from the basic propositions of MHIM2 to predict Generation-separated levels of Severity in the women is virtually the same as its power to predict MH, 12 percent and 11 percent respectively.

The life-span model derived from the basic propositions of MHIM2 fails to predict Generation-separated Severity in the men, although it had predicted nine percent of their levels of Generation-separated MH. The only prediction is that the Earlier Generation of the men has a more favorable Generation-separated average level of Severity than does the Later Generation (AC, IC, and AIC).

* * *

We have seen that the life-span model derived from the basic propositions of MHIM2 does not predict levels of some other 1974 adult functioning outcomes as well as it predicts MH74. However there are some notable variations:

- The model predicts the following about as well as it does MH74: level of Affective Symptoms in 1974, Generation-separated level of Affective Symptoms among the Midtown women, and increase in level of Severity of Somatic Disorders between 1964 and 1974.
- The model fails to predict among the Midtown men the levels of 1954 Affective Symptoms, Generation-separated Affective Symptoms, Affective Episodes, and Generation-separated Severity of Somatic Disorders. Among the Midtown women the model fails to predict only the level of increase in Severity of Somatic Disorders between 1954 and 1964.
- The model predicts the following at a substantially lower level than it does MH: 1954 levels of Affective Symptoms, in the panel and in the women; increase in level of Severity of Somatic Disorders from 1954 to 1964, in the panel and in the men; level of Generation-separated Severity of So-

matic Disorders in the panel and in the women; level of Affective Episodes in the panel and in the women; and level of Generation-separated Affective Symptoms in the panel and in the women.

These findings indicate that there are limits to the applicability of the life-span model derived from the basic theorem of MHIM1 associated with the Midtowners' social age (Generation) and Gender, and on the particular outcome measures being predicted.

Notes

1. This description describes in broad measure the findings from extensive use of Pearson correlation and factor analysis. Statistically sophisticated readers are invited to refer to the Statistical Appendices for all of the methodological details and a full presentation of all of the statistical findings described in this chapter.
2. We could not include our analyses of 1974 levels of Income, Education or Occupation in the present monograph due to space limitations.
3. We remind the reader that when the association of a measure with the 1974 measurement of the outcome characteristic, such as level of Affective Symptoms in 1974, is statistically controlled for the 1954 level of that characteristic, e.g., Affective Symptom level in 1954, the resultant prediction is of change in the outcome characteristic, e.g., in Affective Symptom level from 1954 to 1974. Explicit analyses of change in outcome variables from 1954 to 1974 are presented in the Statistical Appendices. They did not yield findings meriting space in the present monograph.
4. The references in chapter 3 addressing SES as a "fundamental cause" of impaired health status are relevant here as well.
5. The Generations differ specifically in the numbers falling in the clinically important levels of MH, Well and Impaired. This was explored fully in chapter 7. Generation-separated measures of adult functioning were formed in the same way as GMH.
6. With the expanded access to medical care resulting from the expansion of entitlement programs (Medicaid and Medicare) and health insurance programs in the 1960s, the Midtowners who are 40–59 years of age in 1974 have more medically diagnosed physical health problems in 1974 than the Midtowners who were 40–59 years of age in 1954 had in 1954. The possibility must be acknowledged that there may have been an attrition from the panel of Midtowners who in 1954 were 40–59 years of age and who had unfavorable levels of somatic disorders; i.e. some physically ill Earlier Midtowners may not have survived to be part of the MHIM2 panel.

9

Predictions of Mental Health from Personal History Derived from the MHIM2: Expected versus Observed

We have undertaken in the last five chapters of this monograph to explore the most fundamental theorem of MHIM in longitudinal perspective: aspects of sociocultural contextual settings (in both their normative and deviant forms) operating both inside and outside of the family, during childhood and adulthood, have measurable consequences reflected in differences in mental health composition among subgroups within a community population.[1] The scientific challenges which we have met, in so doing, involved life-span measures and data analysis: *Measures.* We developed measures of sociocultural contextual settings operating both inside and outside the family during childhood and adulthood by using both the data collected in MHIM1 and some additional items added to MHIM2 to fill in some gaps in the MHIM1 data which became evident to the senior author after the publication of *Mental Health in the Metropolis*. These measures were as follows:

Demographic characteristics: Age level, Gender, Parental Socioeconomic Background.

Contexts of childhood: Three sociocultural measures addressed the family as a microsocial environment for childhood development. We looked at: (1) Parental Intrafamily Functioning, the extent to which the Midtowners portrayed their parents as having created a warm, loving and supportive setting for childhood development; (2) Parental Breadwinner Adequacy, the extent to which the Midtowners portrayed their parents as having reliably and adequately provided for the material necessities and luxuries of life; and (3) Family-Kin Network extensivity, the extent to which the Midtowners portrayed their childhood family as having social relations with other family members, friends and neighbors in their childhood community. In addition we looked at a biological measure, Body Damage, which differentiated between Midtowners who had basic physical constitutional malformations or malfunctions in their childhood and Midtowners who had sound physical constitutions in childhood.

Pre-Adult Well-Being: This measure was a composite of three biopsychosocial measures of the Midtowners' symptom formation before adulthood: intrapsychic well-being, physical health well-being, and social well-being. It was conceived by the senior author as analogous to adult mental health, but with a pre-adult focus.

Severity of Somatic Disorders Before 1954: This measure summarized the physical health history of the Midtowners up to the 1954 period of measurement of adult mental health in terms of the total level of severity of all somatic disorders which they reported had started prior to 1954, whether in MHIM1 or in MHIM2.

Data analysis. We then were challenged to use these measures to explain in life-span perspective the 1954 adult mental health level of the Midtowners. None of the data analytic methods used in *Mental Health in the Metropolis* had statistically modeled the life-span nature of the MHIM1 data. The methods of path analysis, which had become prominent in sociological methodology by 1969, became known to the senior author and his colleagues as adequate for this purpose.

Essentially path analysis begins with the overall associations between a characteristic such as adult level of mental health and the other measures included in a model of that characteristic, such as Sociodemographic Background, Contexts of Childhood, Pre-Adult Well-Being, and Severity of Somatic Disorders up to 1954. The overall associations are sequentially adjusted for each type of other measures in the model, arrayed by the segment of the life cycle they address, to yield predictions, e.g., of adult level of mental health.

These predictions embody the life-span nature of the MHIM1 data. We must remember, however, that the data collection was not longitudinal but, rather, cross-sectional. All of the data was collected at the same time, but, for example, some of the data referred to the biosocial background of the Midtowners, some to the characteristics of their family settings in childhood and adolescence, and some to their level of functioning as adults in 1954. The path analyses bring out the life-span nature of the periods of the life cycle to which these cross-sectional data refer.

The 1974 data collection, however, broke new ground: all of the MHIM1 data was collected twenty years earlier, so that the longitudinal nature of the relationship between the MHIM2 data and MHIM1 data was intrinsic, not simply a matter of assumptions made in constructing statistical models. As specified in the senior author's research plan, the fundamental theorem of MHIM1 was extended in longitudinal perspective to formulate the basic propositions of MHIM2.

The decision to use path analysis eventuated in the junior author's joining the MHIM2 research team as a statistical researcher in 1976. We have described in general terms the findings of multiple path analyses of adult mental health (MH) in 1954 in this monograph, and shall make our final summary below. There were three types of sequences in which the overall associations of measures in the model with 1954 MH were corrected for other types of measures in the model, as follows:

Intervening, Concurrent (IC): The association of level of Severity of Somatic Disorders up to 1954 and MH54 is also the prediction, because no other measure either comes between these two characteristics in the adult life cycle or occurs reciprocally with Severity. The association of Pre-Adult Well-Being with MH54 is corrected for Pre-1954 Severity to yield an IC prediction. The association of a Context of Childhood, say Body Damage, is corrected for the three concurrent other Contexts (Parental Intrafamily Functioning, Parental Breadwinner Adequacy, and Family-Kin Network extensivity) and for the two measures which intervene between Contexts and MH54, that is, Pre-Adult Well-Being and Severity, to yield an IC prediction. The association of a Demographic measure, say Parental SES, is corrected for the other two Demographic measures, Age level and Gender, and for the intervening types of measures, that is, Contexts, Pre-Adult Well-Being, and Severity, to yield an IC prediction.

Antecedent, Concurrent (AC): The association of level of Parental SES with MH54 is corrected only for the concurrent Demographic measures of Age level and Gender to yield an AC prediction. The association of the level of a Context of Childhood measure, say Body Damage, with MH54 is corrected for the concurrent other Contexts of Childhood measures, and also for the antecedent Demographic measures, to yield an AC prediction. The association of Pre-Adult Well-Being with MH54 is corrected for the antecedent Contexts of Childhood measures and the antecedent Demographic measures to yield an AC prediction. The association of level of Severity of Somatic Disorders up to 1954 is corrected for all of the other measures in the model to yield an AC prediction, for all other measures are antecedent to Severity.

Antecedent, Intervening, Concurrent (AIC): In this sequence the association of each measure in the model with MH54 is corrected for all of the other measures in the model to yield an AIC prediction. The

AIC prediction is the overall association adjusted for all of the associations among the measures in the model. Thus the AIC prediction of MH54 by Pre-Adult Well-Being would be the overall association between MH54 and Pre-Adult Well-Being adjusted for Sociodemographic measures, Contexts of Childhood, and level of Severity of Somatic Disorders up to 1954.

Measures. We proceeded to explore essential research issue of MHIM2: To what extent is the fundamental theorem of MHIM1 substantiated by the life course of the Midtowners up to the 1974 period of measurement? With respect to our primary measure of personal health in 1974, adult level of mental health in 1974, additional measures were introduced into the model of mental health derived from the fundamental theorem of MHIM1 and constituting the basic propositions of MHIM2.

1954 Adult Functioning: The Midtowners had achieved adult statuses outside of their childhood families by the 1954 period of measurement. These included: (1) their 1954 Adult level of Mental Health; (2) their 1954 Own level of Socioeconomic Status (SES54), measured as a composite of their levels of education, occupation, income, and rent; (3) their 1954 level of extensivity of Social Networks, measured as composite of their levels of social relations with family, friends, neighbors, and community residents; (4) their 1954 level of Excess Intakes, measured as a summation of the Midtowners' reports that they drank coffee, smoked tobacco, ate, or drank alcohol "more than is good for you"; and (5) their 1954 level of Affective Symptoms suggestive (but not diagnostic) of depression. To simplify our model of adult mental health derived from the basic propositions of MHIM2, we considered the level of Severity of Somatic Disorders up to 1954 as a measure of 1954 Adult Functioning.

1954 to 1974 Developments: We then looked at four types of developments which, among all of the potential types of developments following 1954, were both associated with level of adult mental health in 1974 and clearly originated in the period preceding the 1974 measurement of adult level of mental health (i.e., were not reciprocal with any adult functioning characteristic in the 1974 period of measurement). These four developments were as follows: (1) Affective Episodes between 1954 and 1974, based on Midtowners' reports that they had periods of unusually high or low spirits affecting their normal routines during this period; (2) Increase in level of Severity of Somatic Disorders between 1954 and 1964, based on the Midtowners' reports that they became aware of these somatic disorders between 1954 and 1964, a ten-year period preceding the overall expansion of the health care service provision and finance system associated with the "Great Society" era; (3) Increase in level of Severity of Somatic Disorders between 1964 and 1974, based on the Midtowners' reports that they became aware of these somatic disorders between 1964 and 1974, a ten-year period including the overall expansion of health care service provision and financing associated with the "Great Society" innovations of Medicare and Medicaid; and (4) Mental Health Treatment, a composite of Midtowners' reports that they had sought professional help for emotional problems between 1954 and 1974 from a variety of mental health practitioners.

Longitudinal data analysis. As in our study of 1954 level of adult mental health, we began by looking at the overall associations between 1974 adult mental health and other measures in the model of adult mental health derived from the basic propositions of MHIM2. We then used path analysis to adjust these associations for each type of other measure in the model, arrayed by the period of the life cycle they characterize, yielding predictions, to yield IC, AC, and AIC predictions. For example, the AC prediction of MH74 by SES54 adjusted the overall association of SES54 and MH74 for the associations among SES54 and other 1954 Adult Functioning measures, which were concurrent, and the antecedent measures including Pre-Adult Well-Being, Contexts of Childhood, and Sociodemographic characteristics. The IC prediction of MH74 by SES54, on the other hand, adjusted the overall association of SES54 and MH74 for the associations among SES54 and other 1954 Adult Functioning measures, which were concurrent, and for the associations with the 1954 to 1974 Developments, which were intervening. The AIC prediction of MH74 by SES54 adjusted the overall association of SES54 and MH74 for the associations among SES54 and all of the other measures in the model of mental health derived from the basic propositions of MHIM2.

Expected versus Observed Predictions

The basic propositions of MHIM2 first imply that aspects of the Midtowners' reported early life experiences are correlated with their biosocial background characteristics. Secondly these propositions imply that both biosocial background characteristics and early life experience are correlated with life outcomes in adulthood, both in 1954 and in 1974. Thus we expect each measure in our model of mental health derived from the fundamental theorem of MHIM to be associated with MH54 and MH74. In chapter 1, we summarized some biosocial measures which were established in MHIM1 to not be associated with adult mental health when the Midtowners' level of parental SES was controlled, specifically Generation in the United States, Religious Origin, and National Origin of Parents. These findings presented MHIM2 with its major hypothesis, which was stated in the form of two basic propositions: (a) Aspects of families' higher or lower positions in their community's socioeconomic structure influence both the personal life of family members with the family and their interactions with other persons outside the family; this creates drastically different settings for children to grow into and out of. (b) These differences begin to influence children's biopsychosocial development during their most impressionable, formative years. Thus we hypothesized that, according to their SES position, parents and the family life setting within which the child grows play a crucial part in the development of the child's vulnerabilities and resistances to mental health risk factors throughout the entire span of the life cycle. We further proposed that these processes may be different for children of each gender, in measurable ways. That is, the life cycle antecedents of adult mental health may be different for the Midtown women than for the Midtown men, reaching back to their early life experience and biosocial background.

All of these basic propositions of MHIM2 were embodied in our path analyses. We will begin by summarizing our findings for adult level of mental health in 1954.

Adult Level of Mental Health in 1954

Expected Predictions

We expected all of the measures in the model of MH54 derived from the basic propositions of MHIM2 to both be associated with MH54 and to predict MH54 independently from their associations with all of the other measures in the model. In having the latter expectation, we were fully prepared to find that some measures would not be observed to independently predict MH54 when other measures are controlled, just as, say, Religious Origin had not been associated with adult level of mental health in 1954 when the Midtowners' level of parental SES had been controlled in MHIM1. To learn as much as possible from exploring the model of mental health, we solved it in the three ways described above (IC, AC, and AIC). In this manner we could see not only the effect of controlling for the Midtowners' level of parental SES but also the effect of controlling for other measures in the model.

Observed Predictions

Measure by measure, this is what we found in the data for the Midtowners overall:

With one exception, all of the measures in the model were observed to be associated in the panel of Midtowners with MH54, as expected. The single exception was level of Extensivity of Family-Kin Networks, which however was associated with MH54 among the Midtown women (but not among the men).

We found, however, the Age level and Gender of the Midtowners could not be simply considered, but rather that the interaction association distinguishing the older women (who were 40–59 in 1954 and 60–79 in 1974) from the younger women (who were 20–39 in 1954 and 40–59 in 1974) and all of the men had to be included in the model, for reasons explained in chapter 4.

When we solved the path model controlling for antecedent and concurrent measures, we observed that AC predictions were made for the Age and Gender interaction, Parental SES, Body Damage, Parental Breadwinner Adequacy, Parental Intrafamily functioning, and Pre-Adult Well-Being, as expected. However, we did not observe the expected AC predictions for Family-Kin Network Extensivity or level of Severity of Somatic Disorders up to 1954. Which associations involving these two measures might have accounted for this departure of the observed from the expected?

First, we remember that Family-Kin Network did not have an overall association with MH54 in the panel of Midtowners. This is itself a departure from expectations based on the basic theorem of MHIM. Recall from chapter 5 that Family-Kin Network itself was predicted by Age level and Parental SES: Older Midtowners had increasingly unfavorable (less extensive) levels of Family-Kin Networks as compared with Younger Midtowners; and Midtowners from increasingly favorable levels of Parental SES had increasingly favorable (more extensive) levels of Family-Kin Networks as compared with Midtowners from less favorable levels of Parental SES. For these reasons we would even more strongly expect Family-Kin Network level to be associated with MH54, but this association was not observed in the panel of Midtowners.

Second, we are reminded that the Midtowners' levels of Severity of Somatic Disorders up to 1954 was consistently predicted by their level of Pre-Adult Well-Being regardless of which statistical controls were used (AC, IC, and AIC). There were also indications that Severity may be predicted by Age level (AC and IC), Body Damage (AC and IC), and Parental Intrafamily Functioning (IC). Our controls for these antecedent measures explain why Severity did not predict MH54. Note however that the control for Parental SES as an antecedent was not pertinent to the lack of an AC prediction of MH54 by Severity. This is the sort of finding that outlines the limits of applicability of the basic propositions of MHIM2 to the prediction of 1954 level of adult mental health, and other outcome measures in this study.

We next solved the path model of MH54 for the IC predictions, finding that, as expected, the Age and Gender interaction, Parental SES, Parental Breadwinner Adequacy, Parental Intrafamily Functioning, Pre-Adult Well-Being, and level of Severity of Somatic Disorders up to 1954 all made IC predictions of MH54. We also observed that the level of extensivity of Family-Kin Networks made an IC prediction of MH54, as expected. No IC prediction was made by Body Damage, due to its association with level of Severity of Somatic Disorders up to 1954. The control for level of Parental SES was not contributory to the insufficiency of Body Damage to make an IC prediction of MH54.

Finally we solved the path model of MH54 for the AIC predictions, finding that, as expected, the Age and Gender interaction, Parental SES, Parental Breadwinner Adequacy, Parental Intrafamily Functioning, and Pre-Adult Well-Being made AIC predictions of MH54. We did not observe AIC predictions for Body Damage, Family-Kin Network extensivity, or level of Severity of Somatic Disorders up to 1954.

Body Damage was not predictive due to its association with the Age and Gender interaction. Family-Kin extensivity lacked an overall association with MH54, and the controls for antecedent measures canceled out the controls for intervening measures. Severity was consistently predicted by Pre-Adult Well-Being, which also consistently predicted MH54. The control for Parental SES was not consequential in any of these variations of observed predictions from expectations.

We continued our exploration of the basic propositions of MHIM2 by analyzing separately the data for the Midtown women and men, and comparing the observations, as follows:

Among the women, all of the measures in the model were associated with MH54. Controlling for antecedent and concurrent measures, predictions were made by Age level, Parental SES, Parental Intrafamily Functioning, and Pre-Adult Well-Being, as expected; but not by Body Damage, Parental Breadwinner Adequacy, Family-Kin Networks, or Severity. In attempting to explain these variations from expectations, we cannot single out any specific controls which resulted in the lack of an AC prediction for Body Damage. Parental Breadwinner Adequacy and Family-Kin Networks were both predicted among the women by both Age level and Parental SES. Severity was consistently predicted among the women by Age level and Pre-Adult Well-Being, but the control for Parental SES was not important in explaining the lack of an AC prediction.

Among the women, IC predictions of MH54 were made by Age level, Parental Intrafamily Functioning, Pre-Adult Well-Being, and level of Severity of Somatic Disorders up to 1954, as expected; but not by Parental SES, Body Damage, Parental Breadwinner Adequacy, or extensivity of Family-Kin Networks. The lack of an IC prediction for Parental SES is central to our exploration of the basic propositions of MHIM2. It is primarily explicable by the control for Pre-Adult Well-Being. Parental Breadwinner Adequacy also predicts the women's level of Pre-Adult Well-Being. The lack of an IC prediction by Family-Kin Networks cannot be attributed to a specific control for an intervening or concurrent measure. Rather we observe that the cumulative effect of controlling the other Contexts of Childhood, Pre-Adult Well-Being and Severity is that Family-Kin Networks did not make an IC prediction of MH54 in the women.

The next step was to solve the path model for AIC predictions of MH54 among the women. Age level, Parental Intrafamily Functioning and Pre-Adult Well-Being all independently predicted the level of MH54 of the women; whereas we did not observe AIC predictions for Parental SES, Body Damage, Parental Breadwinner Adequacy, Family-Kin Network Extensivity, or Severity. We have offered reasons for these variations above. With respect to Parental SES, the controls for Parental Breadwinner Adequacy and Pre-Adult Well-Being made a substantial difference, whereas those for Age, Body Damage, Family-Kin Networks, and Severity did not, either because these measures were not associated with Parental SES or did not themselves predict MH54 in the women.

A basic proposition of MHIM2 implies that the findings among the Midtown women will be different than those among the men. We next turn to the data for the Midtown men:

As with the women, the Midtown men's levels of Parental SES, Parental Breadwinner Adequacy, Parental Intrafamily Functioning, and Pre-Adult Well-Being were associated with MH54, as expected. Unlike the women, the men's Age level, Body Damage, Family-Kin Networks, and level of Severity of Somatic Disorders up to 1954 were not associated with MH54. We conclude that this indicated a limit on the applicability of the fundamental theorem of MHIM to the men in comparison to the women, but this also substantiated a basic proposition of MHIM2.

When we applied our three sets of controls to the life-span model of MH54 in the men, we found that Parental SES consistently predicted MH54 regardless of controls in the men, although among the women only the AC prediction was observed. In both Genders, Pre-Adult Well-Being consistently predicted MH54. But in the men Parental Intrafamily Functioning yielded only an AC prediction, whereas in the women it consistently predicted MH54.

How might we explain variations of observed predictions from expectations among the men? Age level was not associated overall with MH54 among the men, unlike among the women. Parental Breadwinner Adequacy was predicted by the antecedent Parental SES, as was the case in the women. Family-Kin Network extensivity was predicted by the antecedents Age level and Parental SES. It also predicted the men's level of Severity of Somatic Disorders up to 1954. Severity was also consistently predicted in the men by Age level, as in the women; and also sometimes by Parental Intrafamily Functioning (IC) and Pre-Adult Well-Being (AC and AIC). Unlike Parental Breadwinner Adequacy and Family-Kin Network extensivity, Parental SES was not important in explaining the lack of any prediction of MH54 by Severity among the men.

Adult Level of Mental Health in 1974

Expected Predictions

We expected all of the components of the life-span model of adult mental health status in later adulthood (1974) to be associated with MH74. However, we expected that the specific predictions made by various measures would differ for women and men. Indeed this was a basic proposition of MHIM2. Finally we maintained as a heuristic hypothesis that all of the measures in the model of mental health would predict MH74.

Observed Predictions

In the total panel of Midtowners, only Gender, the Age by Gender interaction, Body Damage, and Family-Kin Network extensivity were not associated overall with MH74, a variation from expectation. MH74 was associated with Age level, Parental SES, Parental Breadwinner Adequacy, Parental Intrafamily Functioning, Pre-Adult Well-Being, Severity of Somatic Disorders up to 1954, Social Network extensivity in 1954, Affective Symptoms in 1954, Own level of SES in 1954, MH54, Change in Severity from 1954 to 1964 and from 1964 to 1974, Affective Episodes, and Mental Health Treatment, as expected.

The absence of associations for Gender and the Age by Gender interaction led us to explore gender-specific models of adult mental health level in the Later and Earlier Generations, which we will summarize in the following section. Family-Kin Networks had not been associated even with MH54. Body Damage simply was not associated with MH74 in the panel of Midtowners, although it was among the women.

When we solved the path model of MH74 controlling for antecedent and concurrent measures, we observed predictions for Age level, Parental SES, Parental Intrafamily Functioning, Pre-Adult Well-Being, level of Severity of Somatic Disorders up to 1954, MH54, Change in Severity between 1954 and 1964, Change in Severity between 1964 and 1974, Affective Episodes, and Mental Health Treatment, as expected. However we did not observe AC predictions by Gender, the Age by Gender interaction, Body Damage, Parental Breadwinner Adequacy, extensivity of Family-Kin Network, 1954 Social Network Extensivity, 1954 Affective Symptoms, or SES54.

How might these variations from expectation be explained? Those involving Gender led us to the generational mental health analyses to be summarized following this section. Body Damage was predicted by Age level. Parental Breadwinner Adequacy was predicted by both Age level and Parental SES. Family-Kin Network was not associated with MH74 overall. In analyses which could not be presented in this monograph due to space limitations, Social Network extensivity in 1954 was predicted by Parental SES and Pre-Adult Well-Being, as was 1954 level of Affective Symptoms. Finally SES54 was predicted by Parental SES.

We then solved the path model of MH74 with controls for intervening and concurrent measures, and observed the expected predictions for level of Severity of Somatic Disorders up to 1954, SES54, MH54,

Change in Severity between 1954 and 1964, Change in Severity between 1964 and 1974, Affective Episodes, and Mental Health Treatment. However we did not observe an IC prediction for any Sociodemographic measure, any Context of Childhood measure, Pre-Adult Well-Being, extensivity of Social Networks in 1954, or 1954 Affective Symptoms, as we had expected.

In explaining these variations from expectations, we note that the moderate stability of adult mental health level from 1954 to 1974 is key. We saw that most of the pre-1954 measures predicted MH54. It was not surprising that those that did not predict MH54 would not predict MH74 either. We note that both 1954 extensivity of Social Networks and 1954 level of Affective Symptoms are both associated with MH54 and SES54.

Among the Midtown women, all of the model components except pre-adult extensivity of Family-Kin Networks were associated with their levels of MH74. These fifteen associated model components included levels of Age, Parental SES, Body Damage, Parental Bread-winner Adequacy, Parental Intrafamily Functioning, Pre-Adult Well-Being, Severity of Somatic Disorders up to 1954, 1954 Social Networks, 1954 Affective Symptoms, SES54, MH54, Increase in Severity of Somatic Disorders from 1954 to 1964, Increase in Severity of Somatic Disorders from 1964 to 1974, Affective Episodes, and Mental Health Treatment. However, among the Midtown men a third fewer model components were associated with MH74. The men's eleven associations included levels of Age, Parental SES, Pre-Adult Well-Being, Severity of Somatic Disorders up to 1954, 1954 Social Networks, 1954 Affective Symptoms, SES54, MH54, Increase in Severity of Somatic Disorders from 1964 to 1974, Affective Episodes, and Mental Health Treatment. In brief, the expected associations of model measures were found in the data for the women with but one exception; whereas in the data for the men the number of such exceptions was five.

When the path model of mental health was solved with intervening and concurrent measures controlled (IC), we found in the women that only levels of MH54, Increase in Severity of Somatic Disorders from 1954 to 1964 and from 1964 to 1974, and Affective Episodes made IC predictions of MH74 level. Among the men the IC solution of the path model yielded an overlapping but different set of predictions. As with the women, the men's levels of MH54, Increase in Severity of Somatic Disorders from 1964 to 1974, and Affective Episodes predicted MH74. However unlike the women, the men's levels of Severity of Somatic

Disorders up to 1954, SES54, and Mental Health Treatment also predicted their levels of MH74; and Increase in Severity of Somatic Disorders from 1954 to 1964 did not make an IC prediction of the men's levels of MH74. These findings substantiated the basic proposition of MHIM2 that the life cycle antecedents of mental health in later adulthood would be different for women than for men.

We observed among the Midtown women that when we solved the path model of mental health controlling for antecedent and concurrent measures (AC), predictions were made by the women's levels of Age, Parental SES, Parental Intrafamily Functioning, Pre-Adult Well-Being, MH54, Increase in Severity of Somatic Disorders from 1954 to 1964 and from 1964 to 1974, and Affective Episodes. Among the men, similar AC predictions were made by their levels of Parental SES, MH54, and Increase in Severity of Somatic Disorders from 1964 to 1974. However unlike the women, the men's levels of Severity of Somatic Disorders up to 1954, SES54, and Mental Health Treatment also made AC predictions of their MH74 levels, whereas their level of Increase in Severity of Somatic Disorders from 1954 to 1964 did not make an AC prediction of MH74.

Finally when we looked at which measures would predict MH74 with statistical controls for all other measures (antecedent, intervening, and concurrent [AIC]), we found among the women that only four measures were predictive: MH54, Increase in Severity of Somatic Disorders from 1954 to 1964 and from 1964 to 1974, and Affective Episodes. Again the results for men were overlapping but distinctive: AIC predictions were made by MH54 and Increase in Severity of Somatic Disorders from 1964 to 1974, as in the case of the women; and also by Severity of Somatic Disorders up to 1954, SES54, and Mental Health Treatment; but not by Increase in Severity of Somatic Disorders from 1954 to 1964 or Affective Episodes. The AIC results for women vis-à-vis men supported the basic proposition of MHIM2 that the life-span predictors of levels of mental health in later adulthood would be different for women than for men.

The expansion of access to medical care for the Midtowners in the middle of the sixth decade of this century (Starr, 1982) was a macrosocial influence on our life-span data. It was distinctively associated with the mental health status of the men in comparison to the women. Whereas the mental health status of the women in later adulthood was associated with and predicted by their levels of increase in severity of somatic disorders between 1954 and 1964 and also between 1964 and

1974, that of the men was associated with and predicted by only their level of increase between 1964 and 1974, following the expansion of access to medical care. An important associated finding is that mental health treatment was associated with and predictive of the mental health status in 1974 of only the Midtown men, and not of the women. This suggests that the men entered the mental health treatment arena after 1964, again in conjunction with the expansion of access to health-related services. With greater access to physicians, and also to mental health clinicians ranging from psychiatrists to counselors, Midtowners inevitably received more diagnoses and had their health awareness raised.[2]

Generation-Separated Mental Health

A unique value of MHIM2 is the circumstance that the same measurement of adult mental health status was taken of one group of Midtowners who were 40 to 59 years of age in 1954; and in 1974 of the other group of Midtowners who were 40 to 59 in 1974. This experiment of nature made it possible to study an aspect of the social history of mental health, first by comparing the overall distribution of mental health status in one group of Midtowners who were 40–59 at an earlier time of measurement, 1954, with that of the other group, who were 40–59 at the later time of measurement, 1974. We have called these two groups the Earlier and Later Generations of Midtowners. The primary finding is that the prevalence of impaired mental health was greater in the Earlier Generation of Midtown women as compared with the Later Generation of Midtown women. The prevalence of impaired mental health was about the same in the Later Generation of Midtown women, Earlier Generation of Midtown men, and Later Generation of Midtown men.

We were then able to examine the manner in which the life-span model of mental health derived from the basic propositions of MHIM2 predicted Generation-separated mental health in the total panel of Midtowners, and in the Gender groups separately. Our findings were as follows:

In the total panel of Midtowners, levels of Generation, Gender, Parental SES, Body Damage, Parental Intrafamily Functioning, Pre-Adult Well-Being, and Generation-separated Severity of Somatic Disorders (GSD) were associated with levels of Generation-separated Mental Health (GMH). When we controlled for antecedent and concurrent measures, we found that AC predictions of GMH were made by Generation, Gender, Parental SES, Parental Intrafamily Functioning, Parental Breadwinner Adequacy, Pre-Adult Well-Being, and GSD, but not by the Generation-by-Gender interaction, Body Damage, or Extensivity of Family-Kin Networks. The model controlled for intervening and concurrent measures yielded IC predictions for Generation, Gender, the Generation and Gender interaction, Parental SES, Parental Intrafamily Functioning, Pre-Adult Well-Being, and GSD. With all measures controlled, we observed AIC predictions for Gender, Parental SES, Parental Intrafamily Functioning, Pre-Adult Well-Being, and GSD.

Among the Midtown women, GMH was associated with levels of Generation, Body Damage, Parental Breadwinner Adequacy, Pre-Adult Well-Being, and GSD. Among the men GMH was also associated with levels of Parental Breadwinner Adequacy, Pre-Adult Well-Being, and GSD, but not with Generation or Parental Intrafamily Functioning. Only among the men was GMH associated with Parental SES.

When we examined the findings for the path model of GMH controlling for antecedent and concurrent measures (AC), we found among the women that AC predictions were observed for levels of Generation, Body Damage, Parental Breadwinner Adequacy, Pre-Adult Well-Being, and GSD. Among the men we observed AC predictions also for Pre-Adult Well-Being and GSD but not for Generation, Body Damage, or Parental Breadwinner Adequacy. Again only among the men was Parental SES predictive of GMH.

The path model of GMH with intervening and concurrent measures controlled yielded the following IC predictions in the data for the women: GMH was predicted by Generation, Parental Intrafamily Functioning, extensivity of Family-Kin Networks, Pre-Adult Well-Being, and GSD. In the data for the men GMH was predicted by Pre-Adult Well-Being and GSD, as in the data for the women; but not by Generation, Body Damage, or Parental Breadwinner Adequacy. The IC prediction of GMH by Parental SES was unique to the men.

Finally with all measures controlled, the women's GMH was predicted discretely by their levels of Generation, Parental Intrafamily Functioning, Pre-Adult Well-Being, and GSD, whereas the men's GMH was predicted discretely by their levels of Parental SES, Pre-Adult Well-Being, and GSD.

These findings suggest some of the ways in which the social historical context of the life cycle development of adult mental health status at age 40–59 differed for the Midtown gender groups. These differences, and similarities, contributed to a greater understanding of the basic propositions of MHIM2 in a manner which could not have been foreseen from MHIM1.

Gender-Separated Generation-Separated Mental Health

We end our summary of the findings of MHIM2 with our analysis of the life-span predictors of the single most well-known finding of MHIM2, that the mental health status at age 40–59 of the Earlier generation of women was less favorable than that of the Later generation, which in turn was equivalent to that of both the Earlier and Later generations of men. Would a subset of measures in the life-span model of GMH derived from the basic propositions of MHIM2 help us to understand why this differential distribution of Gender-separated Generation-separated Mental Health had been observed among the Midtowners?

The answer was that there was no strong evidence of such a subset of measures, although of course there was some variation in predictions of GMH in the Earlier and Later generations of men and women. Consistent predictions of GMH were made in both the Earlier and Later generations of women by Parental Intrafamily Functioning and Pre-Adult Well-Being. There was also a consistent prediction made in the Later generation of women of GMH by GSD, and some indication that GSD would predict GMH in the Earlier generation (an IC prediction). Only among the Earlier women was any indication observed that Parental SES might predict GMH (an AC prediction).

Among the men, in contrast, Parental Intrafamily Functioning and Pre-Adult Well-Being were not at all predictive in either generation. GSD was consistently predictive in the Later generation of men, and not at all in the Earlier generation. We also saw that Parental SES was consistently predictive of the Later generation's GMH. The Earlier generation of men were distinguished by the fact that only Pre-Adult Well-Being predicted their GMH.

The Importance of MHIM2

We conclude that MHIM2 demonstrates that aspects of sociocultural contextual settings (in both their normative and deviant forms) operating both inside and outside of the family, during childhood and adulthood, had measurable consequences reflected in differences in mental health composition among subgroups within a community population, specifically the Midtown panel. These consequences differed between gender groups and between groups characterized by gender and generation. MHIM2 is the first study to demonstrate in a community population that the life-span predictors of mental health vary by gender, biological age, and social age. It is also the first study to demonstrate life-span predictors of the consumption of mental health treatment and of the perceived helpfulness of mental health treatment.

We conclude also that the potential for valuable research studies implied by the fundamental theorem of MHIM1 and the basic propositions of MHIM2 remains great, not withstanding all of the material we have presented in this monograph. The life cycle model of adult mental health derived from the basic propositions of MHIM2 suggests some paradigmatic dimensions of individual development, which should be of value in future data collections, with appropriately updated and revised measures.[3]

Notes

1. We restrict this summary exposition to mental health status in earlier and later adulthood in consideration of the space restrictions which have structured this monograph. See the Statistical Appendices for more information.
2. This by no means necessarily benign outcome of medical care has been a principal focus of the recently developing field of clinical epidemiology (Sackett et al. 1985).
3. The usefulness of the MHIM2 model in future developmental psychiatric research is conssitent with, for example, several articles by noted psychiatrist and genetic researcher Kenneth Kendler, M.D. (1986, 1996).

References

Kendler, Kenneth S. "Parenting: a genetic-epidemiologic perspective." *American Journal of Psychiatry* 153 (January 1996): 11–20.

Kendler, Kenneth S. and Lindon J. Eaves. "Models for the joint effect of genotype and environment on liability to psychiatric illness." *American Journal of Psychiatry* 143 (March 1986): 279–89.

Sackett, David, R. Brian Haynes, and Peter Tugwell. 1985. *Clinical Epidemiology: A Basic Science for Clinical Medicine*. Boston MA: Little, Brown and Company.

Starr, Paul. 1982. *The Social Transformation of American Medicine*. N.Y.: Basic Books.

Index

Printed and bound by CPI Group (UK) Ltd, Croydon, CR0 4YY

22/10/2024

01777628-0008